The PCOS Thyroid Connection

The PCOS Thyroid Connection

Erica Armstrong, MD, IFMCP

Kelsey Stricklen, MS, RD

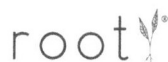

root🌱®
Root Functional Medicine, PLC

CONTENTS

CONTENTS

INTRODUCTION

I wrote this book for women who have struggled with symptoms for months or years without understanding why they were experiencing them and without explanations from health care professionals. Many of these women began to think that the way they feel is just how life is going to be. "Maybe I just need to learn to live with it," they would tell me when we first met at my functional medicine practice.

I'm a medical doctor who spent 8 years as a primary care physician in family medicine. Over the years, women would tell me they are just so exhausted, that their memory isn't as sharp, that their hair is falling out, and that suddenly their skin looked like they were a teenager again. I listened and I saw the pattern. I knew they were telling the truth. All of these women couldn't have possibly been experiencing such a similar constellation of symptoms without reason.

As a conventional doctor, I didn't have as many tools in my tool box as I do now after studying and practicing functional medicine and nutrition. Back then, I would do all the labs I could think of to run, knowing at the time I was ordering them that they would probably come back "normal." Then, my option would be the same option that is often correct on medical board exams: "reassurance."

Unfortunately, these women didn't just want reassurance. They wanted answers. They wanted to feel energy to thrive in their professional and personal lives.

As I learned more in functional medicine, the more everything made sense. Hormone imbalances are very real. Thyroid function can still be a significant factor in how people feel even though labs are in normal ranges (We'll explain more here in this book!). Symptoms like acne and bloating and diarrhea and fatigue are in fact all connected by root causes. Often those root causes are found in the gut and the transformation that happens when the gut heals is remarkable.

I left conventional medicine and went out on my own because I could not ignore the power of functional medicine any longer. I needed to practice this way because it worked and people felt better and it just makes sense to me. I started a small practice and partnered with a dietitian, knowing the power of food and nutrition on health.

The two of us had a passion for PCOS and thyroid at the outset and we've been tracking our members progress, successes in restored hormone balance, fertility, symptom reduction in cravings, fatigue, and even mood over the last three years.

We work in a doctor and dietitian team and the protocols we've developed and refined after treating hundreds of women with PCOS and Thyroid conditions are doable, realistic, and sustainable. We are so excited to share them with you so that you can also achieve these results using the steps in this book.

1

PCOS and Hashimoto's Connection

Throughout my practice as a functional medicine physician specializing in women's health, I helped many women with similar symptoms. Many of these women were suffering from a wide range of symptoms, like digestive issues, brain fog, acne, fatigue, carb cravings, irregular periods, fertility concerns, trouble with sleep, or hair changes. These women had some or all of these symptoms and had different reasons or goals for seeking treatment. Yet, two hormonal conditions causing these symptoms seemed to pop up together quite frequently: polycystic ovary syndrome (PCOS) and Hashimoto's thyroid disease.

While seemingly affecting very different parts of the body, these two conditions continue to show up in pairs in many of the women I treat. What is the connection between these two unique disorders?

If you've picked up this book, then chances are you are one of the number of women who may have polycystic ovary syndrome, thyroid disease, or both. The first half of this book aims to review the unique connection and similarities between PCOS and Hashimoto's thyroid disease and break down the root causes so that you can begin to find your own root cause.

The second half of this book will provide you with our proven 3-month system to begin to reverse these conditions. Unlike many other functional medicine books, we did not want to advertise a "30 day cure," "30 day Challenge," or "30 day Plan." What you will learn in this book is sustainable for a lifetime, because it is realistic and it works beyond 30 days and the 3 months we have outlined. Resetting hormone balance by treating the root cause issues is a journey and this method will help you take control in a way that you will achieve and continue to achieve. The lifestyle habits developed over the 3 months become easier to follow, and as we have seen in our practice, can completely reverse symptoms.

The 3-month plan described in this book is very similar to the program we use for our individual members of our practice all over the country. It is tried, tested, and backed by evidence-based research. The approach we use is called functional medicine, which simply means that we investigate and optimize the body's function by respecting that the body works together as an intricate system and not isolated organs or body parts.

What is Functional Medicine?

You are unique. You have your own genetic makeup, health history, and lifestyle. Your treatment plan should be unique to you too. Functional medicine is an approach to treating health conditions and preventing disease by finding the root cause of your health issues. However, instead of stamping you with a diagnosis and only treating your symptoms, functional medicine doctors find out *why* you have the diagnosis. They will do an in-depth assessment to look at all of your body systems (not just the one causing symptoms), and evaluate how well your body is communicating. Then, functional medicine doctors will recommend interventions to help restore balance by addressing factors such as nutrition, movement, stress, sleep, and gut health.

Functional nutrition is a powerful cornerstone to functional medicine. It uses food as a natural medicine to help restore balance, replete nutrient deficiencies, heal the gut, and more.

Personalization is the main difference between functional and conventional nutrition.

Functional nutrition focuses on the patient instead of the disease. It is a personalized method of optimizing your health based on your individual genetics, lab values, lifestyle, and more. There are no generic meal plans or handouts, because each individual person is different! Functional nutrition honors the fact that food is not only fuel for your body, but also an extremely useful tool to help us address the underlying cause of your condition. A functional medicine dietitian may recommend certain anti-inflammatory foods, gut-healing compounds like glutamine or probiotics, or targeted supplements to replete any nutrient deficiencies based on lab testing.

When you identify and treat the root causes of your hormonal imbalances, you will find that your body works like a beautiful symphony. This book will show you how to start loving your body and working with it, not against it.

What is PCOS?

Polycystic ovary syndrome (PCOS) is one of the most common hormonal disorders affecting women of reproductive age and is the leading cause of female infertility in the United States. Depending on the criteria for diagnosis, PCOS may affect up to 20 percent of all women, although an estimated 70 percent of women with PCOS may be undiagnosed (1). As suggested in the name, polycystic ovary syndrome is a reproductive disorder that involves enlarged ovaries that may house multiple cysts. For women in their reproductive years (typically ages 15-49), the ovaries produce and release an egg into the reproductive tract at the midpoint of the menstrual cycle each month. This is known as ovulation. The ovaries are also responsible for producing reproductive hormones like estrogen, progesterone, and to a much smaller degree, testosterone.

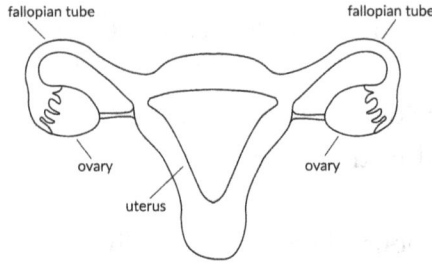

Female anatomy: The egg starts in the ovary, travels down the fallopian tube, and if fertilized, implants in the uterus.

While the name may lead you to believe that PCOS only affects the ovaries, it actually involves your whole endocrine (hormone) system as well. In fact, the main hormones involved in PCOS are insulin, which is made in the pancreas, and testosterone. Imbalances in these two hormones can lead to typical PCOS symptoms for which women often seek medical care: irregular periods, acne, facial hair growth or thinning hair on the scalp, and infertility. Some women may also have cysts on their ovaries; however, this is not necessarily required for a PCOS diagnosis.

There are a few significant risk factors that increase your chances of developing PCOS like having a family history of the condition, or a diagnosis of type 1, type 2, or gestational diabetes. Due to hormonal imbalances, a history of weight gain often occurs before developing other signs of PCOS. While weight may increase your risk of PCOS, research shows that the effect is very modest. For example, one study found the risk of PCOS between normal-weight and overweight women—based on body mass index (BMI)—only varied by 0.1 percent (1). Ultimately, there is much more to this complex condition than the number on a scale.

Signs and Symptoms of PCOS

PCOS is classified as a syndrome and not a disease, which is partly why it may seem so confusing. Nonetheless, most women with PCOS will ultimately seek medical care related to four common complaints: irregular periods, acne, facial hair growth or thinning hair on the scalp, or infertility. Yet, PCOS encompasses a broad spectrum of clinical signs and symptoms that many women may not even realize.

Table 1 shows common signs, symptoms, and health conditions that women with PCOS may experience. The estimated percent of women with PCOS affected by these conditions is reported as well (1).

Table 1

Sign, Symptom, or Condition	Percent of Women with PCOS
Insulin Resistance	50-70%
Impaired Glucose Tolerance	30-40%
High Blood Pressure	22%
Hirsutism (unwanted hair growth)	Up to 70%
Alopecia (thinning hair on the scalp)	16%
Acne	15-30%
Infrequent Periods	85-90%*
Absent Periods	30-40%*
Infertility	40%
Depression	35%
Anxiety	13-63%
Bipolar Disorder	11-27%
Binge-Eating Disorder	12%
Polycystic Ovaries	83-97%

*For clarification, in the women reporting infrequent periods, an estimated 85-90 percent of them will have PCOS while 30-40 percent of women with absent periods will have PCOS.

This list is not exhaustive of all possible symptoms seen in PCOS and many of these conditions are intricately connected. For instance, insulin resistance can often lead to weight gain or difficulty losing weight. Consequently, this weight gain can worsen other clinical signs like high blood pressure or high cholesterol.

Diagnosing PCOS

The most common criteria used to diagnose PCOS is the Rotterdam criteria. This is a list of three criteria that have shown to accurately capture the women who have PCOS.

For a definitive PCOS diagnosis, women must meet at least **two** of the following three criteria:

- Clinical and/or biochemical hyperandrogenism (hair loss on head or hair growth on face, hormonal acne)
- Infrequent ovulation or absence of ovulation (which leads to irregular or absent periods)
- Polycystic ovaries

In order to confirm a PCOS diagnosis, your health provider must exclude any other potential causes of absent ovulation or hyperandrogenism, like thyroid disease, Cushing's syndrome, hypothalamic amenorrhea, and androgen-producing tumors. Let's discuss each of the PCOS diagnostic criteria in more detail.

Clinical and/or Biochemical Hyperandrogenism

Androgens are sex hormones present in both men and women but with higher concentrations found in men. The main androgens include testosterone, androstenedione, and dehydroepiandrosterone sulfate (DHEA-S). In women, androgens are produced by the ovaries, adrenal glands, and fat cells.

When a woman's body produces too many androgens, known as hyperandrogenism, the resulting clinical symptoms are usually dermatological in nature: acne, excessive facial or body hair (hirsutism), or thinning hair on the scalp (alopecia). Hyperandrogenism is present in about 60 to 80 percent of PCOS cases (2).

While clinical symptoms alone often hint at hyperandrogenism, confirming excess androgens with a blood test allows for further investigation. To test for hyperandrogenism, your health provider may order a blood test including total serum testosterone and DHEA-S. In our practice, we often look at additional functional testing, like the DUTCH test, which can also show metabolism of these hormones and additional hormones.

There are no universal reference ranges for these blood tests, so each laboratory may have different cutoffs for what is considered normal. We'll discuss androgen testing more in chapter four.

Infrequent Ovulation or Absence of Ovulation

The menstrual cycle is a natural hormonal change that occurs monthly in women during their reproductive years. It begins with the onset of bleeding typically referred to as your period or menstruation. We call the first day of menstrual bleeding day one of your monthly cycle. Around the midpoint of your menstrual cycle, an ovary releases an egg into the reproductive tract—this is known as ovulation. If the egg is not fertilized by a sperm cell, the lining of your uterus will eventually shed which triggers bleeding and the beginning of your next menstrual cycle. From beginning to end, a healthy menstrual cycle typically lasts between 24 and 35 days.

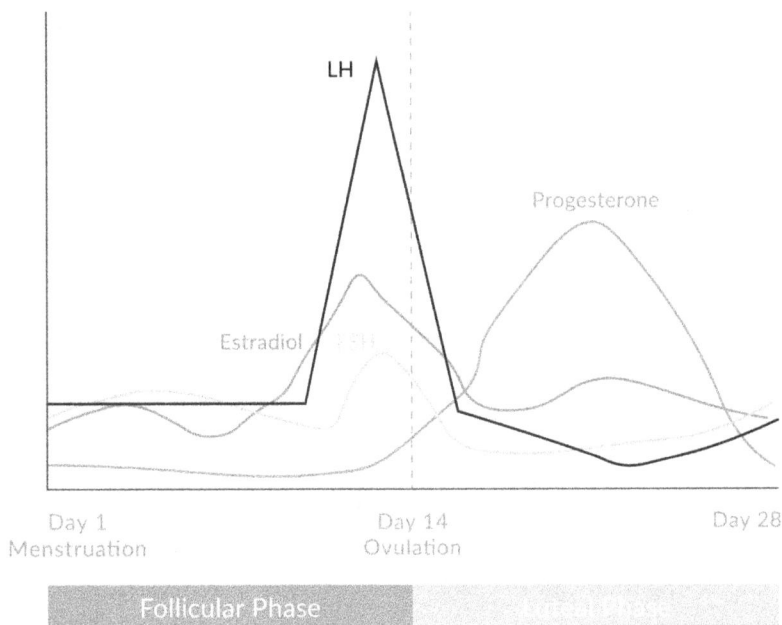

LH

Progesterone

Estradiol

Day 1
Menstruation

Day 14
Ovulation

Day 28

Follicular Phase

Day 1 is the first day of menstrual bleeding, which is shedding of the lining of the uterus. After this, follicle stimulating hormone (FSH) from the pituitary gland in the brain signals the next cycle to begin and estrogen starts rising, preparing the next egg to be released and the uterine lining to thicken again to prepare for implantation. Once estrogen is high enough, FSH stops being released and luteinizing hormone (LH) is released from the pituitary. LH stimulates ovulation if the egg is ready. After ovulation, the corpus luteum is made in the ovary, which produces progesterone in the second half of the cycle. If the egg is not fertilized and implanted, progesterone production stops, triggering the period (menses).

Cycle length can vary due to temporary situations like illness, travel, or stress. However, women with PCOS often have menstrual cycles longer than 35 days due to infrequent or absent ovulation. In fact, an estimated 85 to 90 percent of women who report infrequent periods actually have PCOS.

Nonetheless, it's important to note that the Rotterdam criteria do not *require* irregular periods or ovulatory dysfunction for a diagnosis of PCOS. This is important because up to 30 percent of women with PCOS actually have normal periods.

Polycystic Ovaries

During a normal menstrual cycle, a small number of egg cells begin to grow in the ovary. These are called follicles. The biggest and most dominant follicle will eventually rupture and release the egg from the ovary to trigger ovulation. In women with PCOS, hormonal imbalances often prevent these follicles from maturing and releasing an egg for ovulation. As a result, the leftover follicles in the ovary form cysts frequently seen in PCOS cases.

Occasional ovarian cysts are actually quite common and rarely pose any serious health problems. However, the presence of *multiple* cysts on the ovaries is the third Rotterdam criteria for a PCOS diagnosis. Polycystic ovaries are diagnosed with a vaginal ultrasound device by counting the number of follicles per ovary. In the ultrasound report, the "cysts" of PCOS are often called "follicles." This is the more anatomically correct term, however, many women are unaware that they actually have polycystic appearing ovaries because the report lacks "cyst" in the results. The latest thresholds indicate the presence of 19 to 25 follicles per ovary are indicative of polycystic ovaries and tend to form the characteristic string of pearls stuck on the ovarian wall seen in PCOS (2).

Conventional Treatment Strategies

Conventional treatment of PCOS depends on the symptoms reported and typically fit into three treatment categories: androgen-related symptoms, menstrual cycle irregularities, and infertility. A conventional health provider may prescribe certain medications to help manage these symptoms and/or recommend general weight loss.

Unfortunately, conventional medicine usually fails to treat the root cause of PCOS and leaves most women feeling frustrated and stuck inside the vicious cycle of managing symptoms and side effects.

This book will further discuss and compare conventional versus functional medicine treatment of PCOS in chapter two.

What is Hashimoto's Thyroiditis?

Hashimoto's thyroiditis is an autoimmune thyroid disease involving chronic inflammation of the thyroid gland.

Your thyroid is a small, butterfly-shaped gland at the front of your neck that produces two important hormones: tetraiodothyronine (T4) and triiodothyronine (T3). These thyroid hormones influence essentially every organ in the body and have an enormous effect on health. For example, the thyroid gland helps to regulate bodily functions such as (3):

- Resting heart rate
- Basal metabolic rate
- Respiratory rate
- Body temperature
- Red blood cell production
- Folate and B12 absorption
- Gastric tone and motility
- Fetal growth
- Menstrual cycle
- Growth and development

To carry out these important jobs, the pituitary gland in your brain "tells" your thyroid how much hormone to produce by releasing thyroid-stimulating hormone (TSH). If more thyroid hormones are needed, your brain will release more TSH. If fewer thyroid hormones are needed, your brain will release less TSH.

When stimulated by TSH, the thyroid will produce mostly T4 thyroid hormone and only a small amount of T3. Your T3 hormone is actually considered the "active" version of thyroid hormone that the body can use. However, most T3 is created in the liver and gastro-intestinal tract by converting T4 into the active T3 version. Figure 3 illustrates the cascade of events leading to the development of thyroid hormones.

TSH from your pituitary gland tells the thyroid to produce mostly T4 and a little T3. T4 gets converted to the active form, T3, in your tissues: mostly the liver and intestines. Certain factors, like stress and inflammation, cause T4 to get converted into Reverse T3 (RT3) instead. RT3 is "the brakes." RT3 (the brakes) and T3 (active form) then compete to enter the cell to either produce energy or not.

With Hashimoto's thyroid disease, the immune system mistakenly attacks the thyroid gland causing progressive damage and inflammation. Over time, your thyroid is unable to produce adequate levels of T4 or T3. This gradual decline in function eventually leads to a thyroid condition known as hypothyroidism.

Hashimoto's is the most common cause of hypothyroidism in the United States. While around 5 to 10 percent of the general population suffers from Hashimoto's, women are 10 times more likely to have this disease than men (4).

Signs and Symptoms of Hashimoto's

Because Hashimoto's eventually causes hypothyroidism—an "under-active" thyroid—most of the common signs and symptoms of this disease correlate with symptoms of hypothyroidism. If Hashimoto's is caught early, some people may only have one or two symptoms because the thyroid damage is not significant enough to reduce thyroid hormone production yet.

People with Hashimoto's disease may experience the following:

- Constipation
- Brittle nails
- Dry skin
- Thinning hair or hair loss (alopecia)
- Weight gain
- Difficulty losing weight

- High cholesterol
- High blood pressure
- Fatigue
- Slow heart rate
- Muscle cramps
- Cold intolerance
- Depression
- Heavy or irregular periods
- Infertility

Diagnosing Hashimoto's

Diagnosing Hashimoto's involves one or two simple blood draws to look at a few key hormone and antibody levels.

If you report one or more symptoms of thyroid disease, your health provider will likely first order a blood test to look at your TSH and free T4 levels. A high TSH with or without a low free T4 first confirms the presence of hypothyroidism. Currently, there is a discrepancy in what is considered normal for TSH and what is considered optimal.

TSH Conventional range 0.5 - 4.5
TSH Optimal range 1.0 - 2.5

Typically, the conventional range for a normal TSH level is approximately 0.5 - 4.5 mIU/L. However, functional medicine practitioners often prefer a narrower and more optimal range for TSH of 1.0 - 2.5 mIU/L. Using this smaller range helps to identify more thyroid problems because individuals with a TSH greater than 2 mIU/L have an increased risk of both hypothyroidism and Hashimoto's (5)

The additional presence of thyroid antibodies in your blood indicates the body's immune system is attacking the thyroid gland. Your doctor may include these antibody tests in the initial thyroid panel, but most conventional providers only order additional testing once hypothyroidism is confirmed.

There are two specific antibody blood tests to identify Hashimoto's. First, thyroid peroxidase antibodies (TPO Ab) are immune cells that indicate the immune system is attacking the enzyme in the thyroid gland responsible for producing thyroid hormones. This is the most common target of attack for Hashimoto's. Secondly, thyroglobulin antibodies (TGB Ab) are immune cells that indicate the immune system is attacking thyroglobulin—the precursor to thyroid hormone in the thyroid gland. This is the second most common target for Hashimoto's disease. Both of these antibody levels will be high if you have Hashimoto's.

Unfortunately, many cases of Hashimoto's are missed because providers are using conventional TSH ranges and/or do not test for thyroid antibodies. Occasionally, TSH and T4 can be normal even in the presence of positive antibodies. If you suspect a thyroid issue, it is important to request a *full* thyroid panel to include:

- TSH
- Free T4
- Free T3
- Thyroid Peroxidase Antibodies (TPO Ab)
- Also nice to have: Thyroglobulin Antibodies

Conventional Treatment Strategies

Conventional treatment of Hashimoto's is relatively straight-forward with a goal of closely replicating normal thyroid function by prescribing thyroid hormone. This medication is known under the brand name of Synthroid or generically as levothyroxine.

Your doctor will typically give you a blood test 6 to 8 weeks after you begin taking thyroid hormone and adjust your dose as needed. There are some exceptions to this treatment regimen. For example, people with elevated thyroid antibodies but normal TSH and free T4 levels are not always treated with thyroid hormone replacement. In this case, conventional treatment may only include occasional monitoring of thyroid hormone blood levels and symptoms.

This book will further discuss and compare conventional versus functional medicine treatment of Hashimoto's thyroid disease in chapter two.

The PCOS and Thyroid Connection

Polycystic ovary syndrome (PCOS) and Hashimoto's are two of the most common hormone disorders affecting women.

Around 15 to 20 percent of women have PCOS while an estimated 5 to 10 percent of the general population has Hashimoto's thyroid disease. However, women are 10 times more likely to have Hashimoto's than men and up to 9 percent of women develop Hashimoto's after pregnancy (6).

As the rates of both PCOS and Hashimoto's disease increase, the connection between the two conditions are becoming more recognized. For instance, women with PCOS are three times more likely to also suffer from Hashimoto's thyroid disease than women without PCOS. More specifically, one study found that Hashimoto's was present in 23 percent of women with PCOS versus only one percent of women without PCOS (7). Another larger study found Hashimoto's thyroid disease in 27 percent of women with PCOS compared to only 8 percent of similar-aged women without PCOS (8).

Similarities Between PCOS and Hashimoto's

Now that you know more about PCOS and Hashimoto's individually, let's review the similarities and the most common signs and symptoms that tend to overlap between these two conditions.

Polycystic Ovaries

Polycystic ovaries are one of the most intriguing clinical signs of both PCOS and Hashimoto's. As you know, polycystic ovaries are one of three possible criteria for a PCOS diagnosis. Women with PCOS may develop polycystic ovaries due to hormonal imbalances leading to infrequent ovulation.

In the presence of hypothyroidism, the ovaries may also appear poly-cystic depending on the duration and severity of the underlying thyroid disease. This is why thyroid disorders must be ruled out before making a diagnosis of PCOS.

Menstrual Irregularities

Both PCOS and Hashimoto's can cause irregular menstrual cycles. PCOS causes infrequent or absent periods due to high levels of androgens, like testosterone. Likewise, women with thyroid disease are also more likely to experience infrequent periods and/or heavy periods.

Unfortunately, PCOS and Hashimoto's are also associated with higher rates of infertility, which is defined as an inability to conceive after at least 12 months of unprotected intercourse. A staggering 40 to 50 percent of women with PCOS and/or Hashimoto's experience infertility (1, 9). Women with either of these conditions are also twice as likely to experience early pregnancy loss, which is a miscarriage in the first trimester (9, 10).

Insulin Resistance

Another underlying similarity between PCOS and Hashimoto's is the insulin resistance often found in both of these conditions. Insulin is a hormone released by your pancreas that helps to balance blood sugar levels, among other things. Insulin's main job is to take sugar out of the blood and drive it into the cells that need sugar for energy. Insulin resistance occurs when insulin is unable to enter your cells to take sugar in with it, consequently leading to high levels of insulin and glucose (sugar) in your blood.

Unfortunately, insulin resistance may also cause weight gain or increased difficulty in losing weight, a common occurrence in both PCOS and Hashimoto's. We will further discuss insulin resistance and its effect on the body in chapter three of this book.

Other Common Symptoms

Mood disorders and hair loss or thinning of the hair are two other clinical features that women with one or both of these disorders may experience. Refer to Figure 4 for an illustration summarizing many of the similarities discussed between PCOS and Hashimoto's.

PCOS and Hashimoto's

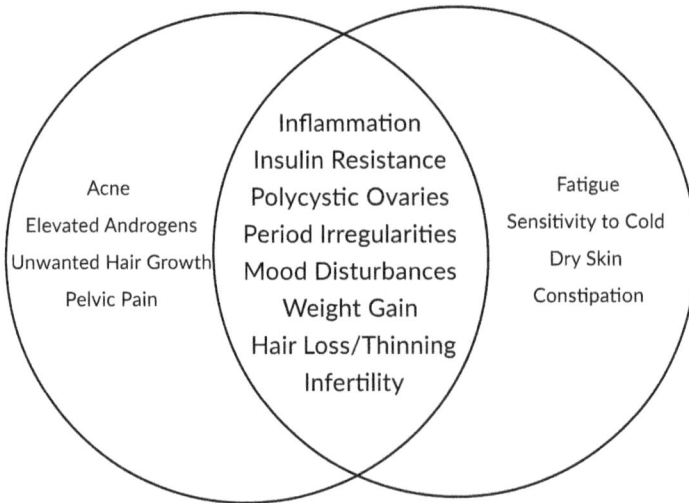

Acne
Elevated Androgens
Unwanted Hair Growth
Pelvic Pain

Inflammation
Insulin Resistance
Polycystic Ovaries
Period Irregularities
Mood Disturbances
Weight Gain
Hair Loss/Thinning
Infertility

Fatigue
Sensitivity to Cold
Dry Skin
Constipation

Key Takeaways

- Polycystic ovary syndrome (PCOS) is diagnosed when you meet at least two of the following three criteria: excess androgens (like testosterone), infrequent or absent ovulation, and polycystic ovaries.

- Hashimoto's thyroid disease is an autoimmune disorder that is diagnosed when you have high levels of thyroid antibodies in your blood with or without an elevated TSH and a low T4 level.
- Women with PCOS are three times more likely to also have Hashimoto's thyroid disease.
- PCOS and Hashimoto's both lead to similar signs and symptoms like polycystic ovaries, irregular menstrual cycles, insulin resistance, and mood disorders.

Getting to the Root Cause

Modern medicine has made tremendous advances in the past century. Discoveries of medications, like antibiotics, prevent death from serious infections every day. Conventional medicine has an important place in our world when treating acute injuries and conditions like a broken bone, appendicitis, or serious bacterial infections, like sepsis. However, conventional medicine often fails to properly address and treat chronic conditions, like PCOS and Hashimoto's thyroid disease. In this chapter, we'll discuss the typical treatment of PCOS and Hashimoto's, review the potential downsides, and explain why treating these conditions with a root cause approach will give you much better and longer-term outcomes.

First, let's discuss the typical treatment of PCOS which fits into three categories: treatment of androgen-related symptoms, treatment of period irregularities, and treatment of infertility.

Conventional Treatment for Androgen-Related Symptoms

Hyperandrogenism, or excess androgens, is one of the three diagnostic criteria used for PCOS. Remember, androgens are hormones like testosterone, DHEA-S, and androstenedione. Excess androgens are responsible for many common symptoms of PCOS, such as hirsutism (excessive or abnormal hair growth), alopecia (thinning or loss of hair on the scalp), and acne.

In conventional medicine, an oral contraceptive—the birth control pill—is typically recommended first for the treatment of androgen-related symptoms in PCOS. Birth control pills can reduce androgens by

1. telling the ovaries and adrenal glands to make fewer androgens;
2. increasing sex-hormone-binding globulin (SHBG), a protein that binds to androgens and decreases their effects;
3. reducing the conversion of a highly potent androgen called di-hydrotestosterone (DHT) from testosterone (1).

The second treatment option for androgen-related symptoms in PCOS is anti-androgen drugs, like spironolactone (which is actually a blood pressure medication with lowering testosterone as a side effect). These drugs attach to androgen receptors in your body thereby preventing the androgens from binding and causing negative side effects.

The Downside

We recognize that there are many benefits to conventional treatments of PCOS. For instance, plenty of women experience a reduction in androgen-related symptoms and therefore an improvement in their mental health and overall quality of life. This benefit shouldn't be overlooked! We understand that a woman may choose conventional symptom management for various reasons. However, it's also important to understand the downsides of conventional treatment and recognize that these are not your *only* treatment options if you have unwanted hair growth, hair loss, or acne.

The birth control pill has an important role in preventing pregnancy and allowing women to choose when or if they want to have children. However, there are also various downsides to the pill that most women do not realize, especially when used for purposes other than pregnancy prevention.

First of all, the pill can cause insufficient levels of certain nutrients in your body (2):

- Folate
- Vitamin B2
- Vitamin B6
- Vitamin B12
- Vitamin C
- Vitamin E
- Magnesium
- Selenium
- Zinc

This is a concerning side effect for women with underlying PCOS because most of these nutrients—especially folate, B6, B12, and zinc—are particularly important in optimizing hormone balance. What's more, insufficient levels of these nutrients may also further increase your chances of developing chronic conditions that are already associated with PCOS like insulin resistance, heart disease, and type 2 diabetes. If you are one of the numerous women who have both PCOS and thyroid disease, depletions of magnesium, selenium, and zinc may also have a negative effect on your thyroid health.

Anti-androgen drugs, like spironolactone, may be recommended to women who do not wish to take a hormonal contraceptive but are still experiencing symptoms of excess androgens. However, it is important to note that spironolactone is often prescribed in *combination* with the birth control pill for PCOS related symptoms because taking this drug alone can cause period irregularities and presents pregnancy risks if a woman becomes pregnant while taking it (1).

Conventional Treatment of Irregular Periods

Irregular menstrual cycles are common in PCOS. Many women with this condition report infrequent or absent periods due to infrequent or absent ovulation. Remember, ovulation should occur around the mid-point of the menstrual cycle when an ovary releases an egg into the reproductive tract. Infrequent or absent ovulation causes a longer over-all menstrual cycle and the inside lining of your uterus doesn't "shed" as it should each month. The long-term effects of absent ovulation in PCOS can increase your risk of having an unusually thick uterine lining —called endometrial hyperplasia—and even cancer (3). When your period eventually arrives, you may experience heavy and/or prolonged bleeding.

For this reason, the conventional treatment of irregular periods in PCOS usually involves prescribing a birth control pill or other hormonal contraceptives that can prevent the buildup of your uterine lining. Many of these contraceptives can reduce androgen production in the ovaries, which may reduce androgen-related symptoms as well.

The Downside

Unfortunately, the pill does not actually make your cycle "regular" as often advertised. Rather, it manages PCOS symptoms by reducing the thickening of your uterine lining, preventing ovulation completely, and triggering a "withdrawal bleed" after 28 days. The bleeding that happens on the "blank week" of the pill happens because the hormone was stopped, thus the bleed is a withdrawal from the synthetic hormones in the pill. The bleed you may experience while on the pill is not a regular period, because the uterine lining does not need to be shed at all. This is why women taking the pill may have lighter periods or stop having periods altogether.

Heavy periods, premenstrual syndrome (PMS), and infrequent or absent ovulation usually return once discontinuing the pill. Some women with regular periods before starting the pill even experience what is called "post-pill PCOS." This is usually a temporary condition that leads to infrequent or absent periods for up to a year after discontinuing the pill. Some women with post-pill PCOS may also complain of mild to moderate acne.

Many women also experience negative side effects while taking the pill including:

- Low sex drive
- Vaginal dryness
- Fatigue
- Mood changes
- Nausea
- Breast tenderness
- Headaches or migraines
- Weight gain

Lastly, the World Health Organization states that the use of combined hormonal birth control is contraindicated for women with high blood pressure, high cholesterol, or a high risk of heart disease. This is concerning since women with PCOS already have a higher risk of having these conditions. Some studies show that birth control pills can worsen and increase triglyceride levels (a type of cholesterol) by more than 75 percent in women with PCOS (3). While this may be avoided by prescribing a different type of birth control, it is still a concerning side effect to consider.

Conventional Treatment of Infertility

Taking hormonal birth control for PCOS symptom management is obviously counterintuitive if you are trying to get pregnant. Conventional strategies for managing irregular periods and infertility, therefore, follow a different line of treatment. Unfortunately, infertility affects approximately 40 percent of women with PCOS. Infertility is typically defined as the inability to achieve pregnancy after at least 12 months of unprotected intercourse. For this reason, many health providers will not recommend medical interventions for infertility until after this timeline. Although many factors play into fertility, infrequent or absent ovulation is the main cause of infertility in women with PCOS. For this reason, conventional treatments aim to induce ovulation.

Many health providers recommend weight loss as first-line therapy for infertility in women with PCOS who have a BMI greater than 30. A mild weight loss of 5 to 10 percent may increase ovulation, pregnancy rates, and a woman's response to fertility drugs (1).

Clomiphene citrate—or Clomid—is often the first drug of choice for women with PCOS and infertility. Clomid is prescribed to induce ovulation by increasing follicle-stimulating hormone (FSH) from the pituitary gland in the brain. This is the same gland that also releases thyroid-stimulating hormone (TSH). If ovulation cannot be triggered at a gradually increasing rate over six menstrual cycles, the woman is considered to be "Clomid resistant." Likewise, failure to achieve pregnancy after six cycles on Clomid is classified as "Clomid failure." An estimated 15 percent of women with PCOS are considered resistant to this medication (4).

Metformin is another drug that may be used to induce ovulation in PCOS. This drug is typically prescribed to manage type 2 diabetes; however, it may improve ovulation in women with PCOS by increasing the body's sensitivity to insulin, reducing insulin levels, and also reducing androgen production in the ovaries.

The Downside

Clomid is fairly effective at inducing ovulation in up to 80 percent of PCOS patients. However, the pregnancy rate of this drug is about 22 percent per ovulation cycle (4). The drastic difference in these percentages may be due to the negative side effects Clomid has on other important fertility factors. For instance, Clomid can change or "dry up" cervical mucus which reduces the sperm's ability to swim up to the egg for fertilization. In a healthy ovulating cycle, rising estrogen levels signal your body to produce stretchy cervical mucus with an eggwhite consistency. Without enough fertile cervical mucus, the sperm will have a difficult time traveling to the egg. Clomid can also decrease the chances of successful embryo implantation.

There are conflicting opinions regarding the use of metformin to induce ovulation in women with PCOS. While metformin is associated with better pregnancy rates, there is limited evidence that it improves live birth rates when used alone or in combination with Clomid. For this reason, some experts believe that metformin should only be used to treat insulin resistance, glucose intolerance, or type 2 diabetes in women with PCOS—and not as a fertility medication. Metformin can also lead to a vitamin B12 deficiency, alter your gut bacteria, and cause unfavorable side effects like nausea and diarrhea (5).

Ultimately, PCOS is a complex condition affecting many different areas of the body. There is no one cure-all treatment because most conventional treatments are directed at managing the *symptoms* and not the *root causes* of the syndrome itself. Plus, since the pill only masks hormone problems and does not treat the root cause of androgen excess or period irregularities, these symptoms often return with a vengeance after coming off the pill.

Our take: Conventional vs. Functional Treatment of Irregular Periods and Infertility

When we think about the conventional approaches to irregular periods and infertility, it seems like the strategy is to override the hormonal process with the birth control pill and to force ovulation with another medication, such as Clomid. Instead, both issues could be restored by restoring natural ovulation, which is done by restoring egg quality. When a mature, high-quality egg is ready, your body will ovulate that egg. After ovulation, that egg is ready to be fertilized, then implanted in pregnancy. If the egg is not fertilized, the hormone production after ovulation naturally drops and a period happens. The tremendous benefit of restoring periods and fertility by restoring egg quality is that the way we do this also improves the overall health of the woman and potentially the baby as well.

There also is benefit to using both a conventional and functional approach to irregular periods and fertility, and as an MD, I am quite comfortable with that combination.

Conventional Treatment of Hashimoto's

The goal in the conventional treatment of Hashimoto's is to treat hypothyroidism and eliminate related symptoms. Hashimoto's is the most common cause of hypothyroidism—or underactive thyroid—in the United States. When you have hypothyroidism, your thyroid gland does not typically produce adequate amounts of thyroid hormone. Your brain responds to the lower thyroid hormone levels by secreting more and more TSH. As a result, your TSH level will be high.

Treatment of hypothyroidism is straight-forward and typically includes a thyroid medication known as Synthroid or levothyroxine. This medication provides your body with T4 thyroid hormone. Your gut and liver then convert this T4 hormone into the active T3 version that carries out all the important jobs in the body. As a result of providing adequate thyroid hormone through medication, your TSH level should return back to normal range.

However, If you have nutrient deficiencies, poor gut health, or chronic stress, your body's ability to convert T4 into the active T3 version may be impaired, and you may still experience hypothyroid symptoms even while taking medication.

Your doctor will tailor your medication dose based on your TSH levels. As explained in chapter one, the conventional range for TSH is between 0.5 - 4.5 mlU/L. While levothyroxine can sometimes reduce thyroid antibodies (the hallmark feature of Hashimoto's), this is not always the case. The presence of thyroid antibodies is used for diagnosing Hashimoto's in conventional medicine but they are otherwise often ignored.

The Downside

When used in the appropriate dose, thyroid medication has very few side effects. Yet, too much thyroid medication can lower your TSH too much and cause symptoms of hyperthyroidism—or an overactive thyroid. You must take this drug on an empty stomach as some foods and supplements may reduce your body's ability to absorb it. While some individuals may be able to wean off thyroid medication, many people end up taking it for years or even for life.

Because thyroid medication has relatively few side effects, the main downside in the conventional treatment of Hashimoto's is the failure to treat the root cause of the disease. Taking medication may lower TSH into the normal range and reduce some hypothyroid symptoms. However, the question of *why* you developed an autoimmune thyroid condition generally remains unanswered. By ignoring the underlying causes of Hashimoto's, additional health problems can eventually arise. For example, about 25 percent of people with one autoimmune condition end up developing an additional autoimmune disease, like rheumatoid arthritis or celiac disease (6). Additionally, many women will continue to experience symptoms despite taking thyroid medication and/or having a normal TSH level.

Similar to PCOS, Hashimoto's is multifaceted and may have more than one root cause. Inflammation, stress, lifestyle, nutrient deficiencies, poor gut health, and genetics may all be a factor in both PCOS and Hashimoto's.

Treating the Root Causes of PCOS and Hashimoto's

As you can see, conventional medicine is generally a *disease-centered* approach where providers manage a disease based on your symptoms.

In the case of PCOS, typical treatment depends on whether you are reporting symptoms of androgen excess, period irregularities, or infertility. On the other hand, there is only one conventional treatment method for Hashimoto's: prescribing a thyroid hormone medication. If your TSH level is within the conventional range of normal, some providers will not treat this condition at all.

We recognize there are some benefits to conventional treatments of PCOS and Hashimoto's. For instance, many women experience a reduction in symptoms and therefore an improvement in their mental health and overall quality of life. This benefit should not be overlooked and a woman may choose conventional symptom management for various reasons. We also recognize there is a time and place to use medication for Hashimoto's. Thyroid medication can reduce debilitating hypothyroid symptoms while we concurrently address the root cause for a long term solution. We think of thyroid medication more as a replacement of thyroid hormone that your body needs rather than as something to work to eliminate. This is different from medications that override body processes. So, in our practice, we will replace needed thyroid hormone *while* working on root causes.

There is a cost to only managing symptoms. Left untreated, individuals with Hashimoto's may have an increased risk of developing an additional autoimmune disease. Likewise, ignoring the underlying causes of PCOS can lead to worsening symptoms that are increasingly difficult to manage and an increased risk of other chronic conditions like heart disease and type 2 diabetes.

Conventional treatment is not your only option if you have these conditions. Functional medicine is a *patient-centered* and *systems-based* approach that focuses on identifying and addressing the root cause of a disease. Functional medicine practitioners think of the body as a connected and communicating system, rather than a shell containing individual and separated organs. By using a functional medicine approach with PCOS and Hashimoto's, we can identify and address the "why" behind your symptoms. Why are you having infrequent periods? Why are you having difficulty losing weight? What caused you to develop an autoimmune disease like Hashimoto's? With this approach, there are often many "whys" to one condition, as illustrated in Figure 2.1

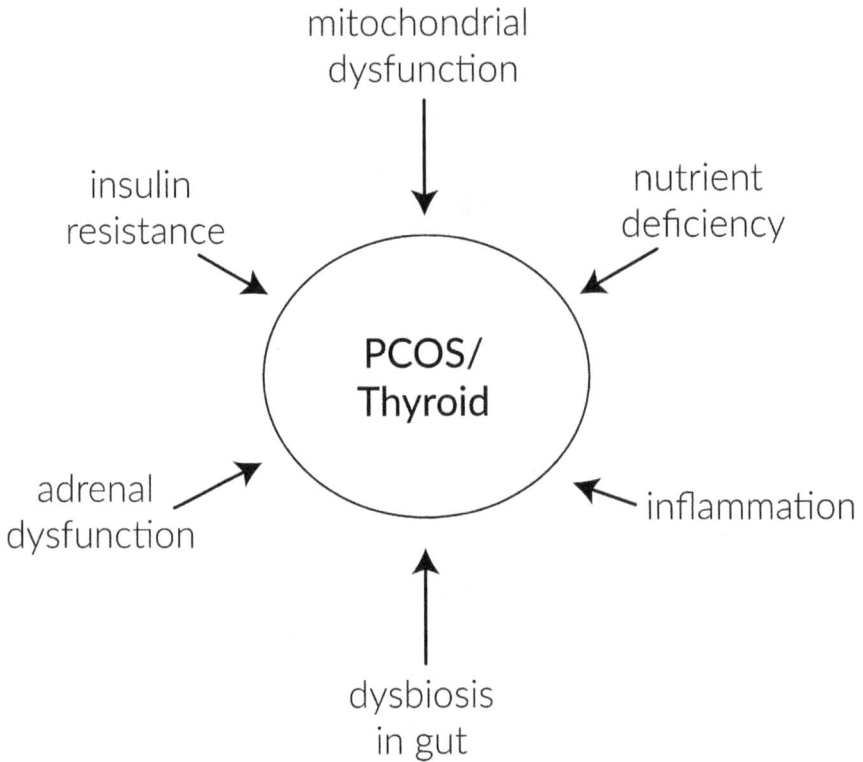

These root causes will be addressed in detail in the following chapters.

Once we identify the root causes or "why" behind PCOS and Hashimoto's, you can begin to reverse these conditions. Yet, the road to healing is not always linear and it is not a sprint. Treating the root cause of chronic conditions like PCOS and Hashimoto's takes commitment. But, the time you spend on your health will pass whether you make the commitment or not. Three months from now, you can look back and be proud of the gradual progress you have made in finding true healing.

Key Takeaways

- The conventional treatment of PCOS depends on your overall symptoms but may include the birth control pill, anti-androgen drugs, metformin, or Clomid.
- The birth control pill does not regulate your period as advertised but rather covers up PCOS symptoms that usually return after discontinuing the pill.
- The conventional treatment of Hashimoto's includes prescribing a thyroid medication to lower TSH levels and reduce hypothyroid symptoms.
- Conventional treatments may reduce symptoms temporarily, but fail to address the underlying causes of PCOS and Hashimoto's. This can lead to more health problems in the future.
- Using a functional medicine and root cause approach, you can identify and address the root causes of both conditions to find true healing.

3

Insulin Resistance

In the first two chapters, we reviewed the signs, symptoms, and conventional treatment methods for PCOS and Hashimoto's thyroid disease. While there are some benefits to these treatments, you may also recognize that conventional methods treat the symptoms and not the root cause. In the next few chapters, we will discuss the underlying causes of these two conditions and provide a brief introduction to the actionable steps you can take to start healing today. In this chapter, we'll discuss the first major root cause of both of these conditions: insulin resistance.

Difficulty losing weight is the number one concern we hear from women applying to work with us. Weight is a primary concern for these women before starting our program for a few reasons. Perhaps conventional medicine has told them for so long that their weight was the cause of their symptoms or PCOS. (**This is not true and we explain to them that difficulty losing weight is a result of having PCOS**). Perhaps they write this because society tells them (even if subliminally) that a lower weight is an indication of health. Or, perhaps they write down their top concern as weight because women with PCOS truly struggle with inability to lose weight due to underlying hormone imbalances, like insulin resistance.

Here is an example case study indicative of so many women we work with in our programs:

Rachel* is a 28-year-old woman who has a history of irregular periods. She was placed on the birth control pill which "regulated" her periods, but she still has many symptoms. Rachel suffers from fatigue, brain fog which worsens after eating, intense cravings for sweets especially 1-2 hours after a meal, and difficulty losing weight. She went on a popular diet that was supposed to last 30 days. She followed this diet for about 17 days and felt great during that time. But, the diet was very hard to sustain with her busy life. As soon as she stopped, she found herself binging on food constantly for the next couple of weeks. She regained the weight she had lost during these two weeks, plus she gained a few additional pounds on top of her baseline weight. She felt so discouraged that she finally reached out to PCOS experts.

*This scenario is not an actual patient, but represents similar situations we treat at Root. Name and age changed for privacy.

We drew an initial lab panel for Rachel which revealed the following:

Fasting Insulin: 9   Optimal Range: Less than 6 µU/mL
Fasting Glucose: 94   Optimal Range: 70 - 85 mg/dL
Hemoglobin A1C: 5.2   Optimal Range: Less than 5.2%

All three of these results indicate insulin resistance. We also found that she was low in vitamin B12, vitamin D, and omega-3 nutrients.

We recommended a nutrition plan for Rachel that was easy for her to follow and realistically sustain with her lifestyle. Her plan did NOT require purchasing various esoteric products from the grocery store. She did not need to spend hours preparing meals ahead of time, and she did not need to bring her separate food to social outings. Instead, she simply developed her own balanced plates using the food available to her with the methods we will talk about in this book.

Another key factor in Rachel's treatment plan was replacing key nutrient deficiencies to help her insulin sensitivity and hormone balance. While long term supplementation is not always needed, Rachel did need some initial supplementation to push her nutrient values to optimal levels.

Finally, we helped Rachel find ways to manage her stress, feel good and confident about her body, and improve her sleep quality. All of these tactics are helpful in balancing hormones and reversing insulin resistance.

Rachel's results were typical of what we see when women follow our plan to reverse insulin resistance. Her cravings were gone and her fatigue improved within a week. By two weeks, her brain fog was starting to clear. By four weeks, she felt in control of her diet and although there were challenges, she used the Root Plate method (see figure 3.3) to stay on track. At three months, we repeated her fasting insulin, glucose, and hemoglobin a1c labs which had all improved significantly. By identifying and addressing the root cause of her symptoms (insulin resistance), Rachel successfully eliminated her symptoms.

What is Insulin Resistance?

Your pancreas makes a hormone called insulin to control blood sugar levels throughout your body. After eating a meal, your pancreas releases insulin into your bloodstream. Insulin essentially acts like a key to open the doors to your cells and allow glucose—broken-down carbohydrates—inside to be used for energy. By moving glucose into your cells, insulin lowers your blood sugar levels back to normal after a meal.

Insulin resistance occurs when your cells do not respond properly to insulin. At this point, there is not anything wrong with the keys (insulin). Rather, the locks on the doors are jammed, making it difficult for the key to open it. As a result, your blood sugar remains high and your pancreas tries to send more insulin in an attempt to normalize blood sugar levels and fuel your cells. Figure 3.1 further illustrates the concept of insulin resistance.

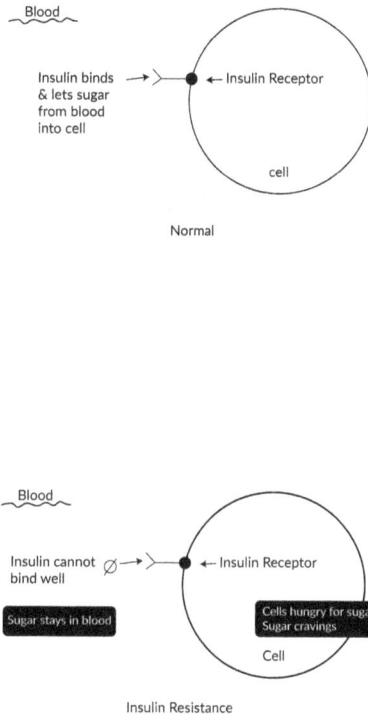

Blood

Insulin binds → & lets sugar from blood into cell

← Insulin Receptor

cell

Normal

Blood

Insulin cannot bind well

← Insulin Receptor

Sugar stays in blood

Cells hungry for sugar
Sugar cravings

Cell

Insulin Resistance

Figure 3.1

If you have insulin resistance, you may experience frequent sugar cravings, fatigue after meals, weight gain or difficulty losing weight, and constant hunger.

Insulin resistance, and elevated insulin levels, is associated with chronic inflammation, hormonal imbalances, ovarian cysts, infertility, and mood changes. As you may have noticed, many of the conditions caused by insulin resistance are common in PCOS and even Hashimoto's, which is why it is vital to address as a significant underlying root cause of these conditions.

Inflammation and Insulin Resistance

Inflammation and insulin resistance have a two-way relationship. Inflammation is your body's way of fighting against infection and injuries in an attempt to heal itself. If you have ever sprained your ankle, you likely noticed swelling as a result of the injury. This type of acute inflammation is helpful and necessary in order to survive. Chronic inflammation, however, occurs when your body's response to injury lingers for a longer period of time. Both PCOS and Hashimoto's disease are associated with low-grade, chronic inflammation. One of the most important tests for measuring inflammation is C-reactive protein (CRP). Unfortunately, women with PCOS have much higher CRP levels than individuals without this condition (1).

Inflammation and insulin resistance create a vicious cycle for women with PCOS and Hashimoto's. Inflammation worsens insulin resistance and insulin resistance causes more inflammation.

Insulin Resistance and PCOS

Up to 70 percent of women with PCOS have some degree of insulin resistance. However, insulin resistance does not only affect women with a higher BMI. In fact, up to 22 percent of women with a normal BMI have been found to have insulin resistance as well (2).

Insulin resistance both directly and indirectly worsens symptoms of PCOS. For example, insulin resistance leads to high insulin levels in the bloodstream and causes the ovaries to produce and secrete more androgens, like testosterone. High androgen levels cause and exacerbate PCOS symptoms like acne, facial hair, and hair loss. Excess androgens also disrupt and prevent proper development of ovarian follicles. When your ovaries cannot release an egg for ovulation, you can experience irregular menstrual cycles, infertility, and polycystic ovaries.

Insulin resistance may also cause weight gain or make it much more difficult to lose weight. This creates a frustrating "catch-22" for women with PCOS because weight loss is often recommended to treat insulin resistance. By shifting the focus on treating insulin resistance instead of prescribing general weight loss, PCOS symptoms improve and women oftentimes lose weight as a positive side effect of treating this underlying cause.

Insulin resistance is concerning not only because of the negative effects it has on PCOS, but also because of what it can lead to if left untreated. Individuals with untreated insulin resistance can eventually develop impaired glucose tolerance (i.e. pre-diabetes) and even type 2 diabetes. Unfortunately, an estimated 30 to 40 percent of women with PCOS already have impaired glucose tolerance and around 10 percent of women with PCOS already have type 2 diabetes (3). We will discuss treatments for insulin resistance later in this chapter and in much greater depth throughout our 3-month plan in the second half of this book.

Insulin Resistance and Hashimoto's

The link between PCOS and insulin resistance is well researched and acknowledged by the majority of medical providers. However, the role of insulin resistance and Hashimoto's thyroid disease is less recognized, even though many studies have been conducted on this topic.

Thyroid hormones affect how your body breaks down sugar. When you have hypothyroidism, your muscle and fat cells become resistant to insulin and do not efficiently allow sugar inside to be used for fuel. This explains why individuals with hypothyroidism often have more insulin resistance and higher insulin levels than people with normal functioning thyroids (4). Plus, if you have both Hashimoto's and PCOS, you may have even higher levels of insulin and insulin resistance than women with PCOS alone (5).

The degree of hypothyroidism has an effect on insulin resistance too. For example, one study found women with PCOS with a TSH level greater than 2 mIU/L had more insulin resistance than women with a TSH less than 2 mIU/L (6). This is yet another reason why we use a functional medicine range of 1 to 2.5 mIU/l when considering optimal

TSH levels. If we allow higher TSH levels, we may be causing other issues like growth of fat cells, increased inflammation, and worsening insulin resistance. See Figure 3.2

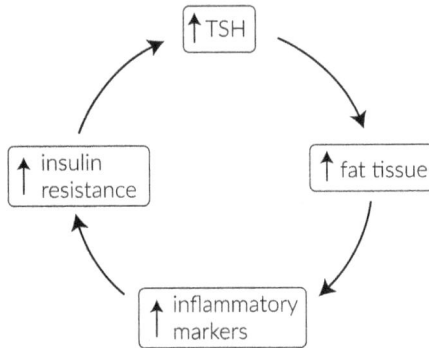

Figure 3.2

Essentially, hypothyroidism causes insulin resistance to some degree. However, inflammation and insulin resistance also worsen thyroid health and symptoms of Hashimoto's.

Inflammation disrupts thyroid health by decreasing the conversion of T4 into the active T3 thyroid hormone. Instead, the body shifts to converting T4 into a hormone called *reverse* T3. Your body requires a delicate balance of reverse T3. Too much of this hormone as a result of low-grade inflammation can slow metabolism, worsen symptoms of hypothyroidism, and cause further hormone imbalances.

Testing for Insulin Resistance

If you have PCOS and/or Hashimoto's, you should consider testing for insulin resistance. Unfortunately, there is no one test that can directly measure insulin resistance. As a result, several tests are often used. Here are a few of the labs we order for our patients to screen for insulin resistance:

Fasting Blood Glucose

This is a measure of how much glucose (sugar) is in your blood after an overnight fast. A fasting blood sugar level between 70 and 85 mg/dL is ideal, and higher levels may indicate insulin resistance. However, we cannot rely on a fasting blood glucose level alone.

Hemoglobin A1C

Hemoglobin A1c is a blood test that measures your average blood sugar levels over the past three months using a percentage point. An ideal a1c level is below 5.2 percent, while higher levels may indicate pre-diabetes or type 2 diabetes. While A1C is a helpful tool for an overall picture of your blood sugar levels, solely relying on A1C can significantly under-diagnose insulin resistance.

Fasting Insulin

Insulin resistance is characterized by increased insulin levels in the blood, so we also test for fasting insulin levels to provide a more complete clinical picture. Conventional medicine has a much higher range for what is considered a "normal" fasting insulin level. However, in our practice, we consider an optimal fasting insulin level to be below 6 μU/mL.

C-Reactive Protein (CRP)

An elevated level of CRP in the blood is an indication that inflammation is present in your body. Extremely high CRP levels are seen in acute injuries, like infection, trauma, or surgery. Low-grade inflammation, as often seen in PCOS and Hashimoto's, can cause a mild elevation in CRP. An ideal hs-CRP (or high sensitivity CRP) level should be less than 1 mg/L.

HOMA-IR

The homeostatic model assessment (HOMA) determines insulin resistance with an equation using fasting glucose and fasting insulin levels.

However, some studies show reliance on HOMA-IR as a sole measure may under diagnose insulin resistance and only catch severe cases. For this reason, you may choose to request the other tests first for a better overall picture.

How to Treat Insulin Resistance

Treating insulin resistance as an underlying root cause of PCOS and Hashimoto's can not only eliminate symptoms but also alleviate its consequences, like future development of type 2 diabetes and heart disease. After identifying insulin resistance as a root cause of these two conditions, we must treat it using a multi-pronged approach. This section will briefly review the main strategies for addressing insulin resistance, however, the second half of this book will dive deeper into these specific interventions. It's also important to mention that even if your lab results show no indication of insulin resistance, following these interventions can still help your PCOS and/or Hashimoto's and improve overall health.

Metformin and Insulin Resistance

Metformin is a prescription medication that lowers insulin and fasting blood sugar levels. It is often prescribed to treat insulin resistance and PCOS. Metformin may improve your body's sensitivity to insulin, increase ovulation rates, and reduce androgen levels. Interestingly, metformin has been shown to lower TSH levels in people with hypothyroidism as well. A benefit of metformin is that it does attempt to address insulin resistance as an underlying root cause, which is why some individuals may experience positive results while taking it. However, this drug does have some negative side effects. First of all, taking metformin for longer periods of time may cause a vitamin B12 deficiency. Vitamin B12 has many important jobs in the body like forming red blood cells to prevent anemia, balancing hormones, and optimizing energy levels. What's more, metformin commonly causes symptoms of GI upset like nausea, diarrhea, bloating, and gas. These side effects may be due to metformin's influence on the gut microbiome, and some studies suggest this drug may also cause dysbiosis—an imbalance of gut bacteria.

Eating for Blood Sugar Balance

The food you eat plays a major role in treating insulin resistance and inflammation in the body. In fact, we support using a "food first" approach when addressing insulin resistance. This means that optimizing your overall diet—as in the foods you eat—is foundational in treating PCOS and Hashimoto's.

A diet high in refined carbs, inflammatory fats, and added sugar worsens insulin resistance. These types of foods are also much easier to overeat, which can lead to an overabundance of calories, frequent blood sugar imbalances, and weight gain. On the other hand, an anti-inflammatory diet containing wholesome sources of protein, fat, and fiber improves your body's sensitivity to insulin, balances your blood sugar, and provides the necessary nutrients to optimize hormone function.

Instead of cycling through unsustainable fad diets, focus on a simple formula of protein + fat + fiber for your meals. The Root Plate (Figure 3.3) is a great way to visualize this formula without having to measure out portions or count calories. With this method, half of your plate is full of non-starchy vegetables, up to a quarter of your plate contains a source of complex carbohydrates (think carbohydrates with fiber), and the other quarter of your plate contains a protein source. We also added a visual reminder to include a serving of healthy fats in your meal as well, since fat is foundational in making sex hormones, balancing blood sugar, and keeping you satisfied after a meal.

The Root Plate™

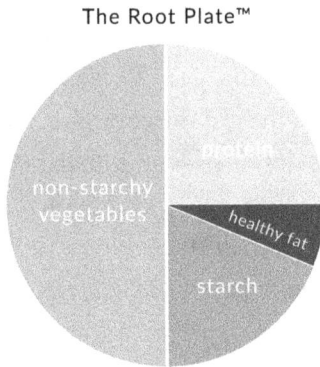

Figure 3.3

For a more detailed list and explanation into this meal planning method, refer to chapter eight.

Improve your Gut Health

The gut is responsible for much more than digestion and nutrient absorption. Believe it or not, the health of your gut also has a major influence on hormonal balance and insulin resistance. Bacteria, viruses, and fungi all collectively comprise a key component of your digestive system—the gut microbiome. Your unique gut microbiome develops over your lifetime and reflects everything about you: how you were born (i.e. vaginally or cesarean section), if you were breastfed, and the various experiences, stressors, diet, and infections you experienced throughout your life thus far. Your microbiome is a complex and ever-changing ecosystem unique to you that can change in response to your environment.

Some of the bugs in your gut microbiome are beneficial to your health, some are harmful, and some are neutral and have little to no effect. When the balance of your microbiome is disrupted, a condition called dysbiosis can occur. Dysbiosis is an imbalance in gut bacteria in which good bacteria are reduced and bad bacteria begin to flourish. Here's where it gets interesting: gut dysbiosis can cause insulin resistance, and women with PCOS and/or Hashimoto's have significantly altered gut bacteria when compared to women without these conditions (7, 8).

To treat insulin resistance, first reduce or avoid environmental factors that lead to gut dysbiosis such as:

- Eating a diet high in added sugar and low in dietary fiber
- Drinking more than seven alcoholic beverages per week
- Inappropriate and/or excessive use of antibiotics
- Regularly taking acid reflux drugs
- Taking hormonal birth control pills (if this is an option)

Since many women with PCOS and/or Hashimoto's may already have dysbiosis, healing the gut is the next step in treating insulin resistance. Healing the gut is much more nuanced than taking a daily probiotic. To improve gut health, we use a functional medicine protocol to first remove any gut infections or dysbiosis, replace missing nutrients, repair the gut lining, reinoculate the gut microbiome, and then rebalance the body for long term success. This strategy is called the 5R protocol.

You will learn more about the 5R protocol in chapter nine of this book.

Balance your Lifestyle

Poor sleep, high stress levels, and a sedentary lifestyle can all worsen insulin resistance.

Approximately one-third of your lifetime is spent asleep. Sleep is necessary for optimal cognitive, physical, and metabolic function. Unfortunately, self-reported sleep times have decreased significantly in the past 50 years and up to 30 percent of Americans report sleeping less than six hours per night. Sleep loss has significant health consequences, especially for blood sugar balance and insulin sensitivity. In fact, poor sleep increases your risk of insulin resistance, elevated glucose levels, and even type 2 diabetes. A simple yet profound intervention you can start today is to aim for seven to eight hours of sleep every night. Reduce sleep disruptors, like alcohol, close to bedtime and avoid drinking caffeine after 1pm. Try establishing a regular bedtime routine now, and we will cover sleep and insomnia interventions more in chapter ten.

High stress levels can also worsen insulin resistance by increasing a stress hormone called cortisol. Cortisol is released from the adrenal glands directly above your kidneys and is required in appropriate amounts to manage blood pressure, inflammation, and your "fight-or-flight" response. However, the demands of modern day lifestyles often cause cortisol to stay elevated for longer periods of time. This can lead to worsening insulin resistance as well as other side effects like weight gain, hormonal imbalances, mood disorders, and insomnia. What can you reduce or eliminate in your life today that is causing unnecessary stress? While it is not often realistic to eliminate all stressors, engage in stress-reducing activities to mitigate the effects it has on your body. Set aside at least 10 minutes of your day for a stress-reducing activity like yoga, meditation, reading, deep breathing, or walking.

Regular exercise is yet another powerful tool that can effectively reverse insulin resistance. Physical activity may promote weight loss, but it also improves your body's sensitivity to the effects of insulin. As a result, insulin can unlock your cells and allow glucose inside to lower blood sugar levels back to normal. A combination of aerobic and strength training appears to be most effective in treating insulin resistance. Nonetheless, the most effective exercise regimen is the one that you will realistically maintain in the long run. Whether this is a 15-minute walk at lunch, or a 30-minute cycling session, set small and realistic goals for including physical activities you enjoy and that make you feel good.

Targeted Supplementation

There is a lot of information out there about the different types of supplements recommended to women with PCOS and Hashimoto's. While many of these recommendations may have well meaning behind them, a lot of them are not evidence-based. The goal of supplementation is not to act as a quick fix for these conditions, but rather to fill the gaps of what may be missing.

However, there are a few supplements for PCOS and Hashimoto's that can generally reduce insulin resistance. For example, inositol is a molecule that may lower insulin levels and improve blood sugar control in women with PCOS. As a result, women with PCOS taking inositol often experience more regular periods, lower testosterone levels, and experience less unwanted hair growth. We recommend taking a 40:1 combination of myo- and D-chiro-inositol to mimic the ratio of the molecules naturally found in the body. Typical doses of myo-inositol in this ratio range from 2 to 4 grams per day. Other supplements found to be helpful in treating insulin resistance may include N-acetyl-cysteine (NAC), magnesium, and fish oil. See the sample supplement schedule appendix for more on dosing.

Key Takeaways

- Insulin resistance occurs when your cells do not respond properly to insulin leading to high levels of sugar and insulin in your blood.
- Insulin resistance drives inflammation which worsens symptoms of both PCOS and Hashimoto's. Insulin resistance also causes an increase in androgen levels, like testosterone.
- Fasting glucose, hemoglobin a1c, fasting insulin, and c-reactive protein are the main blood tests to identify if you have insulin resistance.
- Reversing insulin resistance requires a multi-pronged approach including: eating for blood sugar balance, improving gut health, balancing your lifestyle, and using targeted supplementation when appropriate.

4

Androgens

The next underlying root cause of PCOS and Hashimoto's is hormonal imbalance, namely, high androgen levels. In this chapter, we'll review the different types of androgens, testing, the relationship between androgens and other hormones, and how to achieve hormone balance.

One of the three diagnostic criteria for PCOS is hyperandrogenism. Androgens are sex hormones present in both men and women but with higher concentrations found in men. When a woman's body produces too many androgens, known as hyperandrogenism, she may experience the following symptoms:

- Acne
- Excessive facial or body hair (hirsutism)
- Thinning hair on the scalp (alopecia)
- Weight gain
- Irregular periods
- Irritability
- Insulin resistance

Hyperandrogenism is a chief attribute of PCOS and is present in about 60 to 80 percent of PCOS cases. Interestingly, you may also have higher levels of androgens if you have hypothyroidism.

The Different Types of Androgens

Androgens are produced by either your ovaries or adrenal glands. You have two ovaries—one on each side of the uterus. The ovaries produce and store a woman's eggs and will release an egg when you ovulate. Your ovaries produce about 60 percent of all androgens. You also have two adrenal glands, which are small triangular-shaped glands located on top of both kidneys. The adrenals contribute to about 40 percent of androgen production.

Testosterone

Testosterone is the main androgen in PCOS that is most commonly elevated. It can also be high in certain cases of hypothyroidism. This is another reason it is important to treat both PCOS and hypothyroidism. If only treating PCOS, your thyroid can still contribute to high androgen levels.

About half of your testosterone is made by your ovaries and adrenal glands. The other half is produced by converting androstenedione (a different androgen) into testosterone, which occurs in the liver, skin, and fat cells (1).

In our practice, we measure a total testosterone in a blood lab for every client. However, if there is ambiguity in your diagnosis of progress, there are more ways to evaluate your testosterone level.

Most of the testosterone in your blood is bound to a protein called sex hormone-binding globulin (SHBG) and only one percent is unbound and circulates the blood as free testosterone. Measuring total testosterone levels in addition to SHBG gives us another important ratio called free androgen index. Measuring free androgen index is another way to estimate how much active, or free, testosterone is in your blood.

Reference ranges for testosterone levels vary based on the laboratory running the test and the units used. Below are example reference ranges for what is considered normal testosterone levels for women compared to our goal for optimal testosterone.

Normal total testosterone (Mayo Clinic Laboratories): 8 - 60 ng/dL

Our target range for total testosterone, serum: 20 - 40 ng/dL

Keep in mind, the birth control pill will lower total testosterone, so it's recommended to be off of the pill for at least three months to get a true testosterone level.

Androstenedione

Androstenedione is another androgen that may be elevated in about 18 percent of women with PCOS (2). In women, the adrenal glands and ovaries produce androstenedione, although it does little on its own. Rather, androstenedione is converted to provide about half of your testosterone and almost all of your body's estrone levels—a type of estrogen. The main concern with high androstenedione levels is that it converts into testosterone and can then cause high testosterone levels and symptoms.

Normal reference ranges for women per Mayo Clinic Laboratories: Androstenedione, Serum 30 - 200 ng/dL

Sex Hormone-Binding Globulin (SHBG)

Sex hormone-binding globulin (SHBG) is a protein made by the liver that binds to testosterone in the blood. Women with PCOS generally have lower SHBG levels and therefore higher free testosterone levels. Low SHBG and high testosterone levels are sometimes seen in hypothyroidism as well. By increasing SHBG to the normal range, you can decrease free testosterone levels.

Normal reference ranges for women per Mayo Clinic Laboratories: Sex Hormone-Binding Globulin, Serum 18 - 144 nmol/L

Dihydrotestosterone (DHT)

When testosterone is broken down, dihydrotestosterone (DHT) is formed. However, DHT is more potent than testosterone and much more likely to cause symptoms when elevated. When your body produces too much testosterone, your DHT levels will usually also be high.

The enzyme responsible for breaking down testosterone into DHT is called 5-alpha-reductase. Unfortunately, this enzyme is highly active in women with PCOS and insulin resistance, meaning that these women convert a higher percentage of testosterone into the more potent DHT hormone.

Normal reference ranges for women per Mayo Clinic Laboratories: Dihydrotestosterone, Serum < 300 pg/mL

Dehydroepiandrosterone sulfate (DHEA-S)

Dehydroepiandrosterone sulfate (DHEA-S) is a hormone made by the adrenal glands. While DHEA-S does not do much on its own, it is converted into other powerful hormones like testosterone and estrogen. High levels of DHEA-S are seen in about 25 percent of PCOS patients (2). Stress is a major contributor to DHEA production, and chronic stress can cause high levels of this hormone.

Normal reference ranges for women per Mayo Clinic Laboratories:
DHEA-S 83 - 377 mcg/dL(18 - 30 years)
45 - 295 mcg/dL(31 - 40 years)
27 - 240 mcg/dL(41 - 50 years)
Our goal for DHEA-S for women in the cycling years with PCOS is less than 275 mcg/dL.

DHEA-S is often the only androgen found to be elevated on bloodwork in women with PCOS with an adrenal gland root cause. Chronic internal (stresses within the body like lack of calories or nutrients) or external stress (lifestyle) can send a signal to the adrenal glands to produce both cortisol (the stress hormone) and DHEA-S. We refer to this type of PCOS as adrenal PCOS. See Figure 4.1 We will review this in more detail in the next chapter.

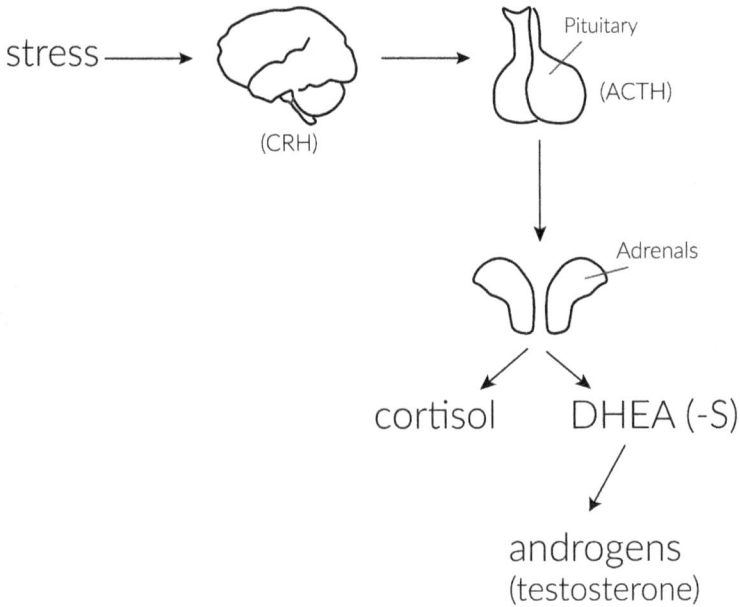

stress⟶ (brain) ⟶ Pituitary (ACTH)
(CRH)

Adrenals

cortisol   DHEA (-S)

androgens
(testosterone)

Figure 4.1

Testosterone and Insulin

Testosterone and insulin have an interesting relationship. Insulin is a hormone made by the pancreas and is responsible for controlling blood sugar levels. We talked a lot about insulin in chapter three. Testosterone is a sex hormone made by your ovaries and adrenal glands. Women need optimal levels of testosterone for bone and muscle strength, sex drive, and estrogen production.

Insulin stimulates the ovaries to produce testosterone. This is a good thing because we need enough testosterone to make another important hormone, called estrogen. However, if you have too much insulin in your blood, the ovaries go into overdrive and make too much testosterone.

Too much insulin also causes the liver to make *less* sex-hormone binding globulin (SHBG). This is the protein that binds to testosterone in your blood. When there is less SHBG to bind testosterone, your free testosterone levels increase. More free testosterone floating around often means worsening acne, unwanted hair growth or hair loss, and irregular periods.

Unfortunately, testosterone and insulin create another vicious cycle for women with PCOS or Hashimoto's, as shown in Figure 4.2. High insulin, as a result of insulin resistance, leads to low SHBG and high free testosterone levels. High testosterone levels in the blood then cause your body to make more insulin, and the cycle continues.

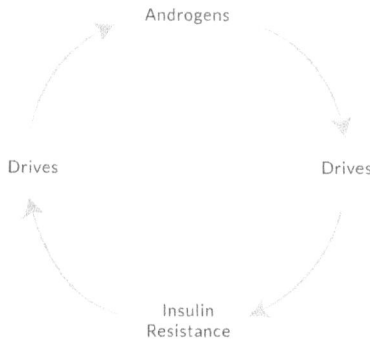

Androgens

Drives   Drives

Insulin
Resistance

Figure 4.2

In order to disrupt this cycle, we have to address what caused the high testosterone and low SHBG levels in the first place: insulin resistance. As you may recall from chapter three, insulin resistance may cause weight gain or difficulty losing weight, sugar cravings, hormonal imbalances, and inflammation. Reversing insulin resistance can reduce testosterone levels and its related symptoms in women with PCOS and thyroid disease.

Testosterone and Estrogen

Estrogen is one of the main sex hormones in women and regulates puberty, your menstrual cycle, and bone health. The ovaries produce most of your estrogen before menopause. However, some of your estrogen also comes from the conversion of androstenedione and testosterone. As a result, women with high testosterone may also have higher estrogen levels (3).

In a normal cycle, your estrogen levels change throughout the month:

- Estrogen levels slowly rise and peak right before ovulation.
- After the ovaries release an egg, estrogen levels drop and progesterone takes over as the dominant sex hormone.
- If your egg is not fertilized by a sperm cell, progesterone levels eventually drop to trigger the beginning of your period.

In PCOS and Hashimoto's, the estrogen fluctuation may not occur because of irregular or absent ovulation. You may have a high or even normal estrogen level. However, without ovulation, your estrogen levels are constantly unopposed because you do not experience the rise in progesterone. This is commonly known as estrogen dominance, or an excess amount of estrogen in relation to progesterone.

Symptoms of estrogen dominance include: weight gain, light or heavy bleeding during your period, mood swings, worsening PMS, and fatigue. Unfortunately, estrogen dominance also seems to increase thyroid antibodies in women with PCOS and Hashimoto's (4).

How to Lower Testosterone Levels

Our 3-month system in the second half of this book will walk you through each intervention to lower testosterone levels and balance other hormones by treating the root cause. Although it may seem overwhelming, many of these interventions overlap with each other! The two main underlying causes of high testosterone levels are insulin resistance and poor adrenal health.

Address Insulin Resistance

If you remember from chapter three, insulin resistance occurs when your cells do not respond properly to insulin, a hormone responsible for balancing your blood sugar. Insulin resistance causes high insulin levels. Higher insulin levels lower SHBG and then raise free testosterone. By normalizing insulin levels and improving your body's ability to respond to insulin, you can lower your testosterone levels. Here are a few basic things you can do to lower insulin levels and reverse insulin resistance:

- Balance your blood sugar by eating an anti-inflammatory diet containing wholesome sources of protein, fat, and fiber with each meal and snack.
- Limit your exposure to environmental factors that can disrupt gut health like excessive antibiotic use, alcohol, and added sugar.
- Get seven to eight hours of sleep each night.
- Incorporate regular physical activity into your routine.
- Consider targeted supplementation like inositol, magnesium, and fish oil.

The best way to know if insulin resistance is one of the root causes of your high testosterone is to request a blood test to evaluate your fasting blood glucose, hemoglobin A1c, and fasting insulin levels. If any of these levels are higher than the normal range, it is likely that insulin resistance is a contributing factor to your symptoms. Refer back to chapter three for more details on these tests and normal reference ranges.

Improve Adrenal Health

Poor adrenal function can be the other underlying cause of your high androgen levels and symptoms. Your adrenal glands make testosterone, androstenedione, and DHEA. While insulin resistance and high insulin levels cause the *ovaries* to make too much testosterone, poor adrenal health causes the *adrenals* to pump out more DHEA and androstenedione. This means that a woman with PCOS symptoms can have normal ovaries (without cysts) and no insulin resistance, but still have symptoms of high androgens.

Stress is the biggest killer of adrenal health. Chronic stress causes the adrenal glands to release more stress hormones and produce excess DHEA. As we discussed earlier in this chapter, about 25 percent of women with PCOS have high DHEA levels. As you consider how to lower stress in your life, think about the root cause approach. What is the root cause of your chronic stress? For some, it may be relationships, finances, or an overextended schedule with too little "me time." It's crucial for your adrenal health that you find a way to identify and lower the root cause of your stress. This may include therapy, talking with a financial advisor, delegating tasks to others, or regularly scheduling time for yourself. However, because stress is a natural part of life, we also need to find a productive way to reduce the effects of everyday stress on our bodies. Set aside at least ten minutes of your day for a stress-reducing activity like yoga, meditation, reading, deep breathing, or walking. We all have at least ten minutes!

A lack of sleep is another stressor to your adrenal glands. Make sure you are practicing healthy sleep hygiene, incorporating regular sleep times, and getting around seven to eight hours of sleep each night.

We will discuss adrenal health, insomnia, and how to heal your adrenals in more detail in chapters five and ten. We will also discuss sources of internal stress, like inflammation, over-restrictive unsustainable diets, and nutrient deficiencies, which can contribute to adrenal PCOS.

What About Supplements?

If you search the internet for "supplements to reduce testosterone", you will find a plethora of blogs, articles, and advertisements touting the health benefits of various supplements promising to reduce testosterone levels in women.

Some of the common supplements recommended include green tea extract, saw palmetto, and zinc. While these may be helpful in reducing testosterone levels to an extent, you must also address the root cause of your high testosterone levels to make any lasting change or improvement. Taking a bunch of supplements and hoping one sticks can cost you a lot of time, money, and energy! Instead, focus on the main root causes of high testosterone: insulin resistance and/or poor adrenal health. Build a healthy foundation of diet and lifestyle and then use supplements to help complement these interventions. For example, inositol helps lower testosterone by lowering insulin and improving your blood sugar levels. Adaptogen supplements, like ashwagandha, may improve adrenal health by balancing your stress hormones.

Don't get caught into the rat race of trying pill after pill to find a fix for your high testosterone symptoms! The way to reduce testosterone for good is not through an "androgen blocker" supplement. It's done by:

- achieving regular ovulation so that the ovaries produce progesterone instead of testosterone,
- decreasing stimulation of the adrenal glands by managing stress,
- and by reversing insulin resistance.

We will discuss targeted supplementation in more detail in the second half of this book.

Key Takeaways

- Androgens are commonly referred to as "male" hormones but are produced by women as well in the ovaries and adrenal glands.
- When your body produces too many androgens, as seen in PCOS and some cases of hypothyroidism, you may experience acne, unwanted hair growth or hair loss, and irregular periods.
- The androgens most commonly elevated in PCOS include testosterone, androstenedione, and DHEA-S.
- The underlying root causes of high testosterone are insulin resistance and poor adrenal health. Treating these conditions can normalize testosterone levels and eliminate many symptoms of PCOS and Hashimoto's.

Adrenal Health

The following story represents the second most common root cause of PCOS and hypothyroidism we see in practice: adrenal dysfunction.

Jennifer* is a 26-year-old graduate student who is planning her wedding. She's concerned that she hasn't had a period for a year. Her doctors keep telling her it's because of stress, but she's had irregular periods since she was 20 years old. They told her she could go on the pill to have a period. However, she knows that taking the birth control pill doesn't answer the question of why she isn't getting a period, and she's concerned about her future fertility. She wants to get to the root cause. She wonders if she has PCOS because she has hair loss, acne, and PMS symptoms. However, her doctors have not suggested that diagnosis.

*This scenario is not an actual patient, but represents similar situations we treat at Root. Name and age changed for privacy.

Technically, Jennifer meets the diagnostic criteria of PCOS with at least 2 out of 3 of the Rotterdam criteria: irregular/missed periods and signs of elevated androgens (hair loss and acne). She may also have cysts on her ovaries, but she hasn't had an ultrasound. In this case, an ultrasound isn't necessary to make the diagnosis, but she may ask her OB GYN for this test if she is curious.

Jennifer's initial lab panel showed the following:

DHEA-S: 430 (high)   Optimal Range 83 - 377 mcg/dL (for 18 - 30 years age)
TSH: 3.5 (high).   Optimal Range 1.0 - 2.5 mIU/L
T3: 2.6 (low)   Optimal Range 3.0 - 3.6 pg/mL

As we discussed in chapter three, DHEA-S is an androgen produced by the adrenal glands. Her high levels of DHEA-S suggests that her adrenal gland is pumping out too much of this hormone. This is likely contributing to her irregular periods, hair loss, and acne. Her TSH and T3 labs fit into a typical "adrenal pattern" as well. For instance, a high TSH is related to adrenal stress and a low T3 stems from an inadequate conversion of T4 (inactive thyroid hormone) to T3 (active thyroid hormone). Stress is a major cause of a poor T4 to T3 conversion. To find true healing, we had to find the source of Jennifer's stress.

As we got to know her daily routine, we find that Jennifer fasts for 16 hours every day, mostly due to running out of the door before having time for breakfast. She found herself working through lunch with just a small snack of hummus and veggies. Jennifer was undereating. This is a significant stress on the body and her brain was telling her adrenal glands, "Send cortisol! We need to store what we have for food." When the adrenal glands release cortisol, they also inadvertently produce DHEA-S.

The first step was helping Jennifer plan a realistic yet balanced breakfast and lunch containing protein, fat, and a fiber-rich carbohydrate. The next step was replacing vital nutrients which are often depleted with stress including B vitamins, vitamin C, and magnesium.

The magnesium greatly increased Jennifer's sleep quality and made it easier for her to wake up on time to eat breakfast. Because her stress had gone on for so long, we also added adrenal adaptogens to her supplement regimen. Adaptogens are herbs that balance cortisol levels and help the body adapt to stress.

Jennifer's root causes took a bit longer to treat. The brain remembers patterns, so it takes consistency to change those patterns. However, after one month, Jennifer is feeling the weight lift from her shoulders. She loves her simple stress reducing techniques that only take a couple of minutes to do. She's happy with her improved digestion and reports experiencing less constipation. She didn't realize her constipation was associated with this hormone imbalance! Now that she is no longer prolonged fasting, she's also including plenty of fiber in her diet.

When we repeated her labs three months later, her DHEA-S was normal at 290, her TSH was within range at 2.5, and her free T3 improved slightly to 2.9. This was a marked improvement achieved with simple lifestyle changes and no medications. Most importantly, she was feeling more like herself and experiencing normal periods by reducing her body's stress.

Stress and PCOS/Hypothyroidism

We mentioned in earlier chapters that adrenal health is another root cause shared by both PCOS and Hashimoto's. We call this adrenal root cause HPA (Hypothalamic-Pituitary-Adrenal) Axis dysfunction. HPA axis dysfunction means that the signal coming from your brain to alert the adrenal glands that there is stress to respond to is not functioning properly. In this chapter, we will narrow in on how your adrenal glands work, how HPA dysfunction affects PCOS and Hashimoto's thyroid disease, and review interventions to achieve hormone balance and symptom relief.

The Hypothalamic-Pituitary-Adrenal (HPA) Axis

The HPA axis is a communication pathway involving your hypothalamus, pituitary gland, and adrenal glands. Your hypothalamus and pituitary gland are located in the brain and your adrenal glands are located on top of each kidney.

- **Hypothalamus:** a pea-sized gland in the brain that acts like a "command center," responding to signals from the body and outside environment to regulate body temperature, hunger and fullness, blood pressure, and hormone production.
- **Pituitary Gland:** a pea-sized gland in the base of the brain that releases important hormones into the bloodstream like prolactin, luteinizing hormone (LH), follicle-stimulating hormone (FSH), and thyroid-stimulating hormone (TSH).
- **Adrenal Glands:** two triangular-shaped glands that sit on top of each kidney and produce stress hormones, like cortisol and adrenaline, and sex hormones like DHEA and testosterone.

In this chapter, we'll focus on one of the main adrenal hormones: cortisol. Although your adrenal glands are the only place where cortisol is made, the communication between the hypothalamus, pituitary, and adrenals is essential to understand and address HPA axis dysfunction as a root cause of both PCOS and Hashimoto's.

Your HPA Axis and Stress

The primary function of your HPA axis is to regulate your response to stress by controlling cortisol levels. While cortisol is normally produced in varying levels throughout the day, the HPA axis regulates what is commonly known as your "fight-or-flight" response.

When you experience a stressful event, your hypothalamus signals your pituitary gland to release a hormone called adrenocorticotropic hormone (ACTH) into the bloodstream. This hormone travels down to the adrenal glands and tells them to release cortisol. The release of cortisol helps your body respond to stress by

- increasing sugar in the bloodstream for your muscles to use for energy;
- suppressing your digestive, reproductive, and immune systems;

- and narrowing your arteries to force blood to pump harder and faster.

If you were in a dangerous situation, these responses help increase your chance of survival. Your body shifts blood and energy to body parts, like your heart and muscles, and suppresses the systems that are not crucial for immediate survival. Who cares about reproduction and immune health when a bear is chasing you? Of course, most people rarely find themselves in recurring life-threatening situations. However, this stress response can also turn on in any experience you may find stressful like public speaking, deadlines at work, or running late for an appointment.

In a healthy HPA axis, the hypothalamus senses high levels of cortisol in the blood and responds by turning down the stress response in what is called a "negative feedback" loop (Figure 5.1). This exists so that your body does not produce excess cortisol when the stressful event is over. In short, your HPA axis was designed to manage short-term stressors.

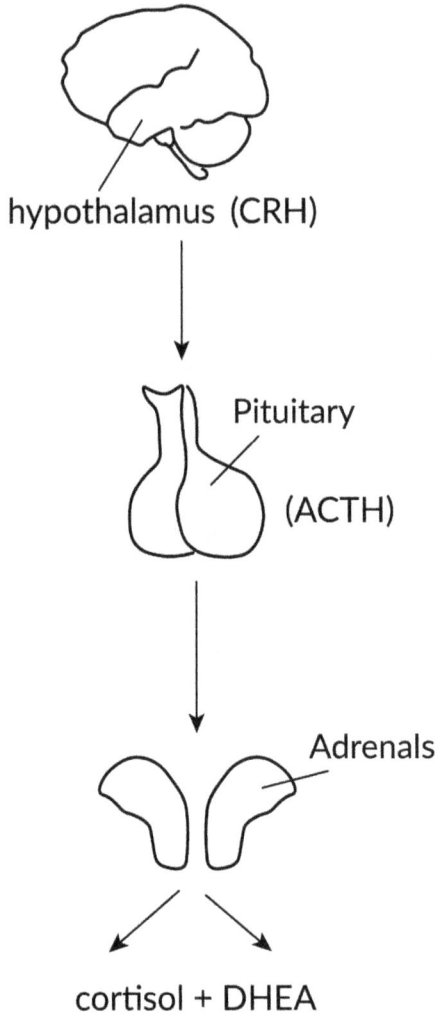

hypothalamus (CRH)

Pituitary

(ACTH)

Adrenals

cortisol + DHEA

Figure 5.1 The HPA Axis

When you live in a state of chronic stress, your adrenals keep pumping out cortisol. Over time, the feedback to your brain can be affected and lead to either high or low cortisol levels.

Symptoms of high cortisol may include: depression, anxiety, insomnia, weight gain, thinning hair, and low libido

Symptoms of low cortisol may include: depression, fatigue, muscle/joint pain, and frequent illness

Is Adrenal Fatigue Real?

Adrenal fatigue is a popular, yet controversial, term often used to describe a wide range of symptoms like brain fog, fatigue, insomnia, and more. Practitioners who support the adrenal fatigue theory suggest that chronic stress drains the adrenal glands and eventually leads to low cortisol levels and the aforementioned symptoms. Most conventional practitioners, however, do not recognize this condition and claim there is no hard evidence to prove its existence. So, is adrenal fatigue real? Yes and no! Your adrenal glands do not stop producing cortisol as a result of chronic stress, but chronic stress can negatively affect the communication pathway of the HPA axis as a whole. However, the issue is likely with the feedback system vs. "fatigued" adrenal glands. For this reason, the more appropriate terminology for this condition is "stress-induced HPA axis dysfunction."

The HPA Axis and PCOS

HPA axis dysfunction is a major root cause of PCOS and is often referred to as adrenal PCOS. In fact, some women do not have insulin resistance or elevated testosterone and only present with signs of adrenal PCOS. Stress, whether emotional or physical, increases cortisol levels. As we read in the story at the beginning of this chapter, stress can also inadvertently increase DHEA-S levels. DHEA-S is an androgen, like testosterone, but is only produced by the adrenal glands. Between 20 to 30 percent of patients with PCOS have high DHEA-S levels (1). Cortisol and DHEA-S disrupt the balance of other hormones in your body that lead to PCOS symptoms like irregular periods, acne, and unwanted hair growth or hair loss. Let's discuss further.

First of all, cortisol raises your blood sugar and decreases your body's ability to respond to insulin (this is called insulin resistance). Up to 70 percent of women with PCOS have some degree of insulin resistance. As we discussed in detail in chapter three, insulin resistance leads to inflammation and increased testosterone levels.

High levels of cortisol may also increase your appetite, trigger sugar cravings, and lead to an increased intake of sugary foods (2). As if this wasn't enough, cortisol triggers your body to store more fat and increases weight gain, especially around the midsection. Weight gain, especially in the belly area, worsens inflammation and insulin resistance as well.

Finally, chronically elevated cortisol levels will suppress the reproductive system. Essentially, this is the body's way of preventing a pregnancy if it perceives a stressful environment that is unfit for pregnancy and reproduction. Through the stress response, high cortisol levels may prevent ovulation or disrupt the hormones needed to successfully conceive and carry a pregnancy to term.

In women with PCOS, we generally see higher cortisol and DHEA-S levels than normal. This happens for a variety of reasons: stress from irregular or absent periods, anxiety due to hormone imbalances, underlying inflammation, erratic blood sugars, or impaired gut health which we will describe in future chapters.

The HPA Axis and Hashimoto's

While Hashimoto's is defined as an autoimmune attack on your thyroid, we can't only blame the immune system. HPA axis dysfunction is one potential cause of Hashimoto's thyroid disease.

Chronic stress and HPA axis dysfunction disrupts thyroid function in a few ways:

1. First, chronic stress causes the adrenals to make more cortisol.

2. The brain senses high cortisol levels and slows down production of active thyroid hormone (T3).

3. Instead of converting T4 into T3, the body shifts into making more of a hormone called *reverse* T3.

4. Reverse T3 turns on the "brakes" and slows down your metabolism.

The body requires a delicate balance of both T3 and reverse T3. Too much reverse T3 as a result of stress and high cortisol slows metabolism and makes hypothyroid symptoms worse. In Hashimoto's and hypothyroidism, we often see high cortisol levels because the body does not effectively break down cortisol (3). Some researchers also suggest that hypothyroidism blunts the negative feedback response of the HPA axis (4). This means that the brain is not responding to high levels of cortisol, and instead of turning down the cortisol release, it tells the adrenals to pump out even more.

Your genetics play a critical role in the likelihood of developing an autoimmune disease like Hashimoto's; however, it is not the only factor. In fact, the autoimmune triad theory Figure 5.2 suggests that in order for an autoimmune disease to develop, one must have genetic susceptibility, environmental trigger(s), and intestinal permeability. Intestinal permeability is the medical terminology for the common phrase "leaky gut." Leaky gut means that the intestinal cell wall is damaged or inflamed and allows large food particles and chemicals through the intestinal wall. We will discuss how gut inflammation and intestinal permeability activate the immune system in chapter seven.

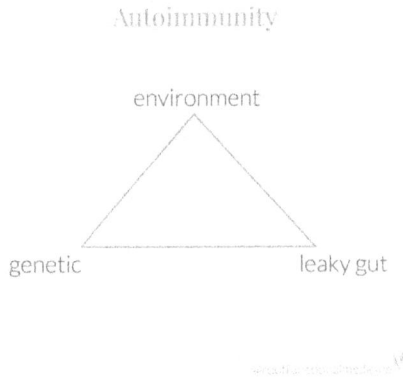

Autoimmunity

environment

genetic   leaky gut

Figure 5.2

Regarding the environment pillar of the autoimmune triad, various environmental factors, like stress or trauma, may increase your chances of developing Hashimoto's. As mentioned earlier in this chapter, your natural stress or "fight-or-flight" response turns down the immune system in order to prioritize systems that are critical to immediate survival. Stress may cause dysregulation of your immune system and lead the body to make antibodies against its own tissues (5).

While we can't do anything about our genetics, we can repair intestinal permeability and control environmental factors, like stress, that lead to autoimmune disease like Hashimoto's.

Our Take: Stress and Root Causes of Hypothyroidism

If you only treat the deficiency of thyroid hormone, as is the common conventional treatment of Hashimoto's, you may still feel symptoms of thyroid disease even if your thyroid numbers are considered "normal." If you continue to feel symptoms of exhaustion, weight gain, irregular periods, and hair loss, yet you're told that your thyroid numbers are normal, you should assess your stress and cortisol levels.

Developing Hashimoto's After Pregnancy

Did you develop Hashimoto's thyroid disease postpartum? Studies show that up to nine percent of all pregnant women develop Hashimoto's after pregnancy. Unfortunately, a Hashimoto's diagnosis after pregnancy is often missed because the related symptoms are brushed off as normal postpartum stress, fatigue, and moodiness. During pregnancy, fetal cells make their way into the mother's blood and may remain there long after delivery. Some researchers believe that this transfer of cells may be the underlying cause of higher autoimmune disease rates postpartum. Stress, HPA axis dysfunction, and abrupt hormonal shifts can also play a role. Whether emotional stress, like postpartum depression, or physical stress, like sleep deprivation, the postpartum period may be an environmental trigger to the development of Hashimoto's in genetically susceptible individuals.

Cortisol Testing

Cortisol follows a circadian rhythm and typically rises quickly upon waking and lowers slowly throughout the day with the lowest point just before bedtime. Cortisol should be at its highest point in the morning to give you energy and lowest before bed so that you can fall asleep. Because of cortisol's rhythmic pattern, testing at only one point in the day does not provide a full picture. Rather, collecting multiple data points throughout the day is the best way to accurately assess your cortisol pattern. For this reason, blood tests are not practical and would require multiple blood draws. However, saliva and dried urine samples offer a practical and accurate method for assessing cortisol patterns (6). When we need to further assess cortisol, we use a four point salivary or urine cortisol testing in our practice. See figure 5.3 for examples of cortisol curves.

Keep in mind that stress-induced HPA axis dysfunction may initially present as high cortisol levels across the day and/or higher than normal levels at nighttime. Over time, the brain may respond by increasing the negative feedback loop, thus leading to low cortisol levels across the board.

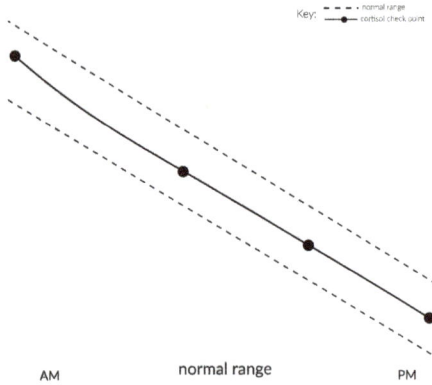

Figure 5.3.1 Normal Cortisol Curve with highest cortisol in the morning, gradually lowering through the day to its lowest point at night.

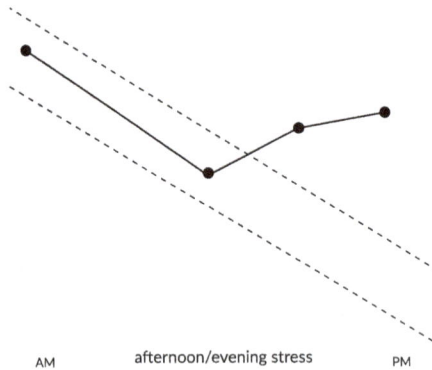

Figure 5.3.2 Cortisol response to afternoon stress. Cortisol starts to rise in the afternoon and stays elevated at bedtime.

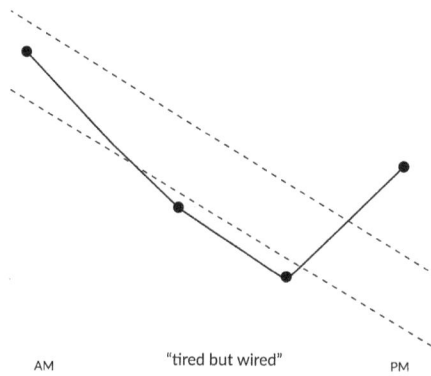

AM   "tired but wired"   PM

Figure 5.3.3 Cortisol curve of someone who may feel "tired but wired." Cortisol is low in the afternoon leading to fatigue, but then spikes before bedtime, making sleep difficult.

Treating HPA-Axis Dysfunction

You will notice that many of the interventions over the past few chapters seem repetitive. That's because they are! This is the beauty of functional medicine. By acknowledging the body as a communicating system, instead of isolated organs, many of the interventions for treating PCOS and Hashimoto's benefit multiple areas of the body and address various root causes.

We dedicated a full chapter to treating HPA dysfunction in the last chapter of this book. But, let's briefly review the main points. Keep in mind that you must address both emotional and physical stressors.

Balance Blood Sugar

Blood sugar fluctuations are a physical stressor that strain your HPA axis. Too much added sugar or refined carbohydrates without enough protein, fat, and fiber will cause your blood sugar to rise and fall dramatically. When you experience what we refer to as the "blood sugar rollercoaster", your body responds by increasing cortisol levels. This rollercoaster is often due to poorly managed meals and snacks.

You may have poorly managed blood sugar levels if you:

- Feel constantly hungry despite eating regularly
- Experience frequent sugar cravings
- Feel "hangry" during the day

You can prevent dramatic blood sugar fluctuations by increasing fiber in your diet, following "PFC" meal guidelines and including a protein, fat, and complex carbohydrate with each meal and snack, and limiting added sugar found in desserts, sweetened beverages, and baked goods.

Improve Gut Health

Inflammation is another physical stressor that can lead to HPA axis dysfunction. Women with PCOS and/or Hashimoto's often have higher levels of inflammation in the body. In order to reduce inflammatory signals that disrupt the HPA axis, we must address poor gut health.

An imbalance of gut bacteria, food sensitivities, and leaky gut can all lead to inflammation and poor gut health. These gut disorders are interconnected and you cannot address one without the other. Healing the gut is much more nuanced than taking a daily probiotic. To improve gut health, we use a functional medicine protocol to remove food sensitivities or gut infections, replace missing nutrients, repair the gut lining, reintroduce probiotics, and then rebalance the body for long term success. This strategy is called the 5R protocol. You will learn more about the 5R protocol in chapter seven and nine of this book.

Stress Reduction and Lifestyle Management

Whether you have high or low cortisol levels, stress reduction and lifestyle management is crucial to healing PCOS and Hashimoto's. In fact, reducing stress may even lower thyroid antibody levels (7). We are often tempted to turn directly to supplements to correct HPA axis dysfunction, however, lifestyle management is arguably the most crucial intervention. **You cannot heal HPA axis dysfunction if you continue to live in a state of constant stress.**

Here are some of the best ways to balance cortisol levels:

- Spend time in nature. Just 20 minutes in nature can lower cortisol levels.
- Implement mind-body practices to center yourself like yoga, prayer, or meditation.
- Optimize your sleep habits by reducing caffeine, eliminating screens before bed, and sleeping in a cool and dark environment.
- Spend time with friends and family. Humans are social creatures and are designed to crave social interaction and connection.
- Invest in therapy to cope with stressful relationships, experiences, or trauma.

Supportive Nutrients and Herbs

While addressing cortisol imbalance with the previous interventions, supportive nutrients, like magnesium, and herbs, like adaptogens, may help your body cope with stress and balance cortisol levels.

Key Takeaways

- HPA axis dysfunction is one root cause of PCOS and Hashimoto's thyroid disease.
- High cortisol levels may cause PCOS by increasing blood sugar levels, worsening insulin resistance, and triggering weight gain.
- High cortisol levels lower active thyroid hormone and increase reverse T3, which can slow metabolism and worsen hypothyroidism.

- The four main interventions for treating HPA axis dysfunction include blood sugar management, improving gut health, stress reduction, and introducing supportive nutrients or herbs.

6

Mitochondrial Dysfunction

In this book so far, you have learned three root causes of both PCOS and Hashimoto's thyroid disease: insulin resistance, high androgens, and HPA axis dysfunction. In this chapter, we will discuss a fourth possible cause of these conditions called mitochondrial dysfunction. You will learn how damage to the mitochondria leads to oxidative stress (and vice versa), the relationship of mitochondrial health to PCOS and Hashimoto's, and how to improve mitochondrial health to treat these conditions and eliminate your symptoms.

If you haven't heard the word "mitochondria" since science class, you're not alone! Let's take a trip down memory lane to review.

What are Mitochondria?

The most common way to describe mitochondria is the "power-houses of the cell," meaning they produce the cell's energy. Cells are the basic building blocks of all living things. Humans are made up of trillions of cells that all work in harmony to carry out basic functions for survival. If you look inside of a cell, you'll see multiple sub-compartments which perform different functions. The main job of the mitochondria is to transform sugar, fat, and protein into energy that the cell can use. This energy, called ATP, cannot be stored. So, the mitochondria must make it every second of every day.

Unfortunately, mitochondria are particularly susceptible to nutrient deficiencies, environmental toxins, and damage from free radicals. Imagine free radicals as little fires that cause damage to your cells. Antioxidants are molecules that protect cells and put out these fires. Oxidative stress occurs when there are too many fires (free radicals) and not enough firefighters (antioxidants). Oxidative stress damages the mitochondria and causes inflammation throughout the body.

Researchers have connected many human diseases with higher levels of oxidative stress including type 2 diabetes, obesity, and insulin resistance. Studies have also shown that women with PCOS or Hashimoto's have higher markers of oxidative stress and lower antioxidant levels than women without these conditions (1, 2).

Mitochondrial Health and PCOS

Sex hormone production starts in the mitochondria. When our mitochondria are damaged, sex hormone production is disrupted which causes hormonal imbalance throughout the body. Mitochondrial damage can also cause derangements in other hormones, like insulin, too. To address the root cause of hormonal imbalance we must address mitochondrial health.

Women with PCOS have significantly higher levels of oxidative stress and lower antioxidant levels than women of the same age and BMI without this condition (1). Oxidative stress can then damage the mitochondria, which may partially explain why women with PCOS are more likely to have conditions associated with mitochondrial dysfunction like insulin resistance, type 2 diabetes, and heart disease. To put it simply: oxidative stress, which damages the mitochondria, is another root cause of PCOS.

When the mitochondria are damaged, they do not function correctly. Mitochondrial dysfunction accounts for several characteristics of PCOS.

Insulin Resistance

An estimated 75 percent of lean women and 95 percent of obese women with PCOS have insulin resistance. Damage to your mitochondria can lead to insulin resistance. As we learned in chapter three, insulin resistance is then largely responsible for the weight gain, weight loss resistance, and the high testosterone levels seen in women with PCOS.

Oxidative stress -> Damage to the mitochondria -> Insulin resistance -> weight gain, weight loss resistance -> high testosterone levels

You need healthy mitochondria for your insulin to function normally. At the same time, healthy insulin signaling is required for optimal mitochondrial function. This creates a tricky "chicken and egg" situation. Do damaged mitochondria cause insulin resistance or does insulin resistance damage the mitochondria? The answer is not simple. Rather, these two scenarios are connected in another vicious cycle. As mitochondria dysfunction and oxidative stress increases, insulin resistance worsens causing even more oxidative stress and damage to the mitochondria!

Impaired mitochondria causes insulin resistance. However, to disrupt the vicious cycle, we must address both insulin resistance and mitochondrial dysfunction to treat the root cause of PCOS.

Irregular Periods and Infertility

Mitochondrial dysfunction may cause the irregular periods and infertility seen in PCOS by either preventing ovulation altogether or decreasing the quality of the ovulated egg.

The eggs in your ovaries have over 100,000 mitochondria each— much more than any other cell in the body. This is because the approximately 90 day period in which an egg slowly develops and matures prior to ovulation requires a tremendous amount of energy. Remember, the mitochondria is responsible for transforming fuel sources into energy your cells can use. Without enough energy, egg development may be deranged or stop altogether. If stopped, your body will not ovulate and the leftover follicles form cysts frequently seen in PCOS cases. This may look like infrequent periods, long cycle lengths, and/or infertility.

If egg development goes awry, the ovulated egg may be more likely to end up with chromosomal abnormalities, the leading cause of miscarriage. Unfortunately, women with PCOS are twice as likely to experience early pregnancy loss, which is a miscarriage in the first trimester (3).

Sperm quality is also an important factor in miscarriage. The quality of the sperm is also affected by the same oxidative stress and mitochondrial health. A traditional sperm analysis in a fertility workup does not thoroughly investigate the oxidative stress in sperm. So, even though your partner may have been told that his sperm is normal, there is still an important role for the male to take in improving fertility. The good news is that there are many reasonable interventions with nutrition, environment and supplementation that you and your partner can do to improve mitochondrial health, and thus egg and sperm quality.

Inflammation

Damage to the mitochondria can cause the chronic, low-grade inflammation seen in PCOS. In addition to higher levels of oxidative stress, women with PCOS also have higher markers of inflammation than women without this condition. This is because oxidative stress eventually causes inflammation. Healthy mitochondria are crucial to control inflammation in PCOS and the other complications connected to inflammation, like insulin resistance and high androgen levels.

Mitochondrial Health and Hashimoto's

Damage to the mitochondria by oxidative stress also has a significant impact on the health of your thyroid. Similar to PCOS, individuals with Hashimoto's tend to have higher levels of oxidative stress than people without this condition (4). In fact, some researchers suggest oxidative stress is one potential cause of Hashimoto's thyroid disease. Oxidative stress also makes hypothyroidism in Hashimoto's worse, and as your levels of oxidative stress increase your symptoms related to hypothyroidism often worsen. As a reminder, common symptoms of Hashimoto's hypothyroidism include:

- Constipation
- Brittle nails
- Thinning hair or hair loss (alopecia)
- Weight gain
- Difficulty losing weight
- High cholesterol
- Fatigue
- Cold intolerance
- Depression
- Heavy or irregular periods
- Infertility

Improving mitochondrial health by reducing inflammation and oxidative stress can help treat this root cause of Hashimoto's and reduce or eliminate many of these symptoms.

Damage to the mitochondria and oxidative stress can cause Hashimoto's; however, your mitochondria also depend on adequate thyroid hormones in order to transform enough energy for the body. When there is a deficiency of thyroid hormones (as seen in hypothyroidism), your mitochondria may struggle to produce enough energy. This may explain why individuals with hypothyroidism often complain of fatigue. We may use medication to correct overt hypothyroidism, even in functional medicine. This may be of particular importance in individuals who have severe cases or may require more immediate treatment (like in the case of hypothyroidism and recurrent miscarriage). We can provide thyroid hormone replacement *and* work towards addressing the root causes of Hashimoto's at the same time. Thyroid medication, or more accurately thyroid hormone replacement, helps restore thyroid hormones to improve mitochondrial function.

It's also important to remember that your T4 thyroid hormone must be converted into the active T3 version in order to enter the cells and drive energy production. If the conversion of T4 to T3 is poor, you may experience hypothyroid symptoms even if you are on medication and/or your TSH levels appear to be normal. Factors that promote the conversion of T4 to T3 include zinc, selenium, lowering stress and inflammation, and optimizing gut health.

Tips to Improve Mitochondrial Health

The diet and lifestyle interventions with the most significant benefit for mitochondrial health are also the ones aiming to reduce overall inflammation and oxidative stress while increasing antioxidant intake.

Eat an Antioxidant Rich Diet

The Standard American Diet (SAD) is rich in calories, inflammatory fats, and refined sugar while lacking in fiber, fruits, and vegetables. Some researchers suggest SAD may trigger autoimmune diseases directly by increasing inflammation, altering the immune response, and modifying the gut microbiome (5). The low intake of fruits and vegetables in a western diet further exacerbates the situation through lower antioxidant levels and worsening oxidative stress. Since mitochondria are particularly susceptible to damage from oxidative stress and inflammation, eating a diet rich in antioxidants is key to protecting these power plants.

The Mediterranean diet is an eating pattern characterized by high intake of vegetables, legumes, fresh fruit, nuts/seeds, whole grains, and olive oil. This diet contains moderate amounts of seafood, poultry and eggs, and lower amounts of red meat and dairy products. The Mediterranean diet is rich in natural antioxidants and has large amounts of research backing it as a powerful anti-inflammatory diet that can also lower oxidative stress.

By increasing your intake of antioxidants from food and limiting inflammatory foods, you can significantly lower your oxidative stress levels and protect your mitochondria from damage.

We will discuss our "food first" plan more in chapter eight. For now, let's review a few common foods that contain some of the highest levels of antioxidants. Start incorporating more of these foods into your diet today!

Common foods containing high levels of antioxidants:

- Berries (all kinds)
- Apples
- Dark leafy greens
- Broccoli
- Asparagus
- Pecans
- Walnuts
- Red kidney beans
- Spices (especially cinnamon, mint, oregano, and thyme)

Red foods, like apples, contain different antioxidants than dark green foods, like spinach. To ensure that you eat a wide variety of antioxidants, aim to make your plate as colorful as possible.

Swap Out Plastics

Bisphenol A (BPA) is a chemical used in various plastic products, like food storage containers, paper receipts, and plastic water bottles. BPA is an endocrine disruptor, which means it interferes with important hormones like estrogen, testosterone, and thyroid hormones. Unfortunately, BPA can also lead to oxidative stress and impair mitochondrial function (6).

Nowadays, most products contain minimal amounts of BPA; however, the ubiquitous nature of BPA unfortunately leads to constant and prolonged exposure for many individuals. Plus, although many products are now "BPA free", manufacturers are simply replacing BPA with closely related chemicals, like bisphenol S.

To reduce BPA exposure, swap your plastic products for glass, stainless steel, or food grade silicone alternatives. Start with the items you use most, like your water bottle and coffee travel mug, and do not microwave your food in plastic containers.

Optimize Vitamin D Levels

Up to 85 percent of women with PCOS have a vitamin D deficiency. Lower vitamin D levels are associated with worsening insulin resistance, period irregularities, and higher androgen levels in PCOS. Similarly, vitamin D deficiency is common in Hashimoto's thyroid disease and treating this deficiency may slow down the development of hypothyroidism (7). Vitamin D supplementation may also improve mitochondrial health by reducing oxidative stress and increasing antioxidant activity (8). Ask your doctor to check your vitamin D levels at your yearly visit. Most labs suggest that normal vitamin D levels are 30 ng/mL or higher and deficiency is 20 ng/mL or lower. However, a "normal level" does not necessarily mean optimal. For our patients, we strive for vitamin D levels around 50 ng/mL for best outcomes.

Vitamin D supplements should be personalized based on your own lab results. For example, if your vitamin D levels are adequate (50 ng/mL), a maintenance dose of about 2,000 units per day may be most appropriate depending on where you live. However, you may require higher doses (5,000 units per day) if your blood levels indicate a vitamin D inadequacy or deficiency. If you are severely deficient, you may require a short term prescription for a megadose of vitamin D.

Omega-3 (Fish Oil)

In addition to vitamin D, omega-3 supplementation can reduce markers of inflammation and oxidative stress while increasing antioxidant levels. Omega-3 fats have also been shown to increase energy production in the mitochondria (9). Fish is the best source of two key omega-3 fats: EPA and DHA. Your omega-3 supplement should contain EPA and DHA for the best outcomes. We often recommend taking about 1,000 mg of total fish oil (EPA + DHA) per day.

Supporting a "food first" mentality, you should also strive to include oily fish into your diet about twice per week. The best seafood sources of EPA and DHA with the lowest amounts of mercury include salmon, mackerel, anchovies, sardines, and herring. You can remember these top five fish by using the acronym "S.M.A.S.H." Fish not only provides you with these beneficial fats but also supports optimal thyroid function through nutrients like selenium and iodine.

Coenzyme Q10

Coenzyme Q10 (CoQ10) is a molecule found in every cell in the body and is critical for energy production inside the mitochondria. It is also an antioxidant that can protect mitochondria from damage and oxidative stress. What's more, CoQ10 supplementation may also lower fasting blood sugar, insulin resistance, and testosterone levels in women with PCOS.

Taking 100 - 200 mg of CoQ10 per day is a great place to start. For best results, take CoQ10 with a meal to enhance absorption.

For recommended supplement products, see the sample supplement schedule in the appendix or rootfunctionalmedicine.com

Intermittent Fasting and Mitochondria

The popularity of intermittent fasting (IF) has grown tremendously over the past few years and many people tout its benefit for mitochondrial health and longevity. There are various methods of IF including alternate day fasting, time-restricted fasting, and periodic fasting. IF may benefit PCOS by promoting weight loss, improving fasting blood sugar, and reducing insulin resistance. While there are some studies also showing anti-inflammatory benefits, research investigating the impact of intermittent fasting on mitochondrial function is limited. A few studies showed no change in mitochondrial health while one reported some protection against oxidative damage (9). Fasting with PCOS and Hashimoto's should be carried out carefully. As always, focus on eating a diet rich in antioxidants, fiber, and fresh foods. Listen to your body, and stop any practice that may make you feel worse, whether mentally or physically. Because of the clear connection between low-calorie diets and reduced thyroid function, we recommend against full-day fasts. A safer alternative may be to extend your overnight fast by eliminating late-night snacking (which tends to involve low-quality foods anyway).

Key Takeaways

- Mitochondria are the power plants of the cell and transform sugar, fat, and protein into energy for your body to use.
- Oxidative stress damages the mitochondria and makes them less efficient at producing energy. Oxidative stress is often the result of diet, lifestyle choices, and/or environmental toxins.
- Mitochondrial dysfunction is one root cause for both PCOS and Hashimoto's and accounts for several characteristics like insulin resistance, period irregularities or infertility, and worsening hypothyroidism.
- You can improve mitochondrial health by eating more antioxidant-rich foods, reducing BPA exposure, optimizing vitamin D levels, eating fish twice per week, and taking a CoQ10 supplement.

Gut Health

Hippocrates said it best nearly 2,500 years ago: "all disease begins in the gut." In functional medicine, we recognize the interconnectedness of the body. Your organs do not work independently of each other. Rather, your gastrointestinal (GI) system, immune system, and reproductive system all function together to optimize human health. When one of these systems is disrupted or imbalanced, it creates a ripple effect impacting other organs as well. If you've ever seen a functional medicine practitioner, you may be surprised at the length and extensiveness of the questions. For instance, if you come to Root for help with irregular periods or a Hashimoto's diagnosis, you will find that we ask you about your bowel habits and digestive symptoms (among many other things). Poor gut health is the last, but arguably most influential, root cause of PCOS and Hashimoto's.

More commonly than not, we see women with PCOS, thyroid, AND gut health symptoms like bloating, constipation, or diarrhea. We find that it is more than a mere correlation for women to have irregular periods and symptoms of disrupted gut health. They are very likely sharing a root cause and that root cause is often found in the microbiome of the gut. Here's a representative case study example (not representing any particular patient, but a common theme we see in our practice):

Jessica* is a 36-year-old woman who came to Root because no one seemed to be putting it all together. She was given birth control for her periods, an antidepressant for IBS (irritable bowel syndrome) with diarrhea and she was still feeling bloated after eating, fatigue, and brain fog. The last straw for her was when her dermatologist wanted to add a daily antibiotic for her acne, which she insightfully knew would likely make her diarrhea worse. She was ready to get to the root cause.

*This scenario is not an actual patient, but represents similar situations we treat at Root. Name and age changed for privacy.

We ordered a functional stool test for Jessica, which is much more detailed than any conventional stool tests. The stool test revealed what we already suspected clinically. Jessica had a dysbiosis (or an imbalance in her microbiome) that was contributing to gut inflammation. That gut inflammation did not stay in her gut; it circulated through the connected blood supply and presented itself in the form of acne, fatigue, brain fog, and anxiety. The dysbiosis was also affecting how her hormones were metabolized and eliminated in the stool. We commonly see this as a source of estrogen and progesterone imbalance.

To help Jessica we placed her on a gut friendly diet, used gentle herbs to rebalance the dysbiosis, targeted probiotics, and a powder blend with nutrients to help heal the intestinal cell lining. She noticed a marked improvement in her brain fog and fatigue first. She was thrilled as she dealt with unexplained fatigue and brain fog for years. Her anxiety lifted shortly into month two. By six weeks, she was noticing improvement in her acne.

Addressing gut health for Jessica not only improved her current symptoms, but may have also prevented the development of autoimmune thyroiditis, or Hashimotos, which we know she was at risk of developing due to her previous diagnosis of PCOS.

A Healthy Gut

When we reference "the gut", we are referring to the stomach, small intestines, and large intestines. However, there are many more key components of your digestive system. A healthy gut is free from inflammation, infection, and dysbiosis or bacterial overgrowth. It contains a bountiful and diverse community of gut bacteria and allows for proper digestion and absorption of nutrients from food.

When you eat or drink, the salivary glands in your mouth release digestive enzymes in your saliva to begin the digestive process. As food travels through your esophagus and into your stomach, the cells in your stomach release acid to break down the food. This stomach acid is particularly important for killing any harmful bacteria from your food as well. Imbalances in the levels of stomach acid may cause intestinal bacterial overgrowth (too little stomach acid) or acid reflux, heartburn, and ulcers (too much stomach acid). The food then enters into your small intestine where most nutrient absorption occurs. Your small intestine moves food along its nearly 22-foot long canal using peristalsis, a wave-like muscle movement to push contents forward. The small intestine is where your pancreas, gallbladder, and liver release more digestive juices, bile, and enzymes to prepare your food for proper absorption. The pancreas also makes insulin and releases it directly into the bloodstream to lower blood sugar levels back to normal after a meal. Your small intestine readily absorbs most of the nutrients from food before it enters into your colon (large intestine). The colon is responsible for absorbing water, digesting fibers, and processing waste to be eliminated through the stool. The colon is also where most gut bacteria should reside. As we will discuss later in this chapter, gut bacteria has a tremendous impact on PCOS, Hashimoto's, and overall health. If the gut has bacterial overgrowth, infection, or inflammation, disease often occurs.

Your Gut Microbiome

The gut is responsible for much more than digestion and nutrient absorption. Bacteria, viruses, yeast, and fungi all collectively comprise a key component of your digestive system—the gut microbiome. Your unique gut microbiome develops over your lifetime and reflects everything about you: how you were born (i.e. vaginally or cesarean section), if you were breastfed, and the various experiences, stressors, diet, and infections you experienced throughout your life. Your microbiome is a complex and ever-changing ecosystem unique to you that can change in response to your environment.

Some of the bugs in your gut microbiome are beneficial to your health, some are harmful, and some are neutral and have little to no effect. Your good bacteria have many important jobs. They maintain a healthy gut lining, prevent overgrowth of harmful bacteria, train the immune system, and make components like vitamins, enzymes, and hormones. When the balance of your microbiome is disrupted, a condition called dysbiosis can occur. Dysbiosis is an imbalance in gut bacteria in which good bacteria are reduced and bad bacteria begin to flourish. Dysbiosis can damage the gut lining, cause food sensitivities, and lead to further disease. In fact, women with PCOS and/or Hashimoto's have significantly altered gut bacteria when compared to women without these conditions (1, 2).

The Gut Lining

Your intestines contain a protective barrier, or lining, to prevent uncontrolled entry of undigested food, bacteria, and toxins from entering the body. It also prevents loss of water and electrolytes while allowing for proper absorption of nutrients. The gut lining consists of your gut microbiome, finger-like villi to aid absorption, and a single layer of cells (Figure 7.1). These intestinal cells are linked together by proteins called "tight junctions" which act as the gatekeepers to control what can or cannot enter the intestinal cells.

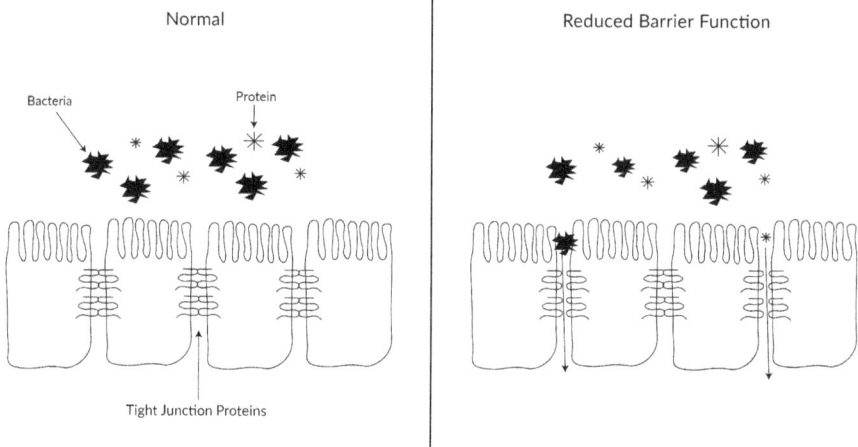

Figure 7.1 Normal gut lining vs. Reduced barrier and disrupted tight junctions.

When the integrity of the gut lining is compromised through dysbiosis, inflammation, or infection, larger food proteins or harmful bacteria may enter into the cell. This is known as a "leaky gut." A leaky gut may cause an unnatural immune response and even trigger auto-immune disease. Some studies also suggest that women with PCOS have higher levels of zonulin, a marker for leaky gut, than women without PCOS (3).

Signs of an Unhealthy Gut

Various factors in your environment may lead to dysbiosis and leaky gut. Antibiotic use, the birth control pill, poor diet, stress, and minimal exposure to bacteria (i.e. the hygiene hypothesis) are just a few factors that may negatively impact your gut health. The hygiene hypothesis suggests that *less* childhood exposure to bacteria may actually *increase* your chances of developing disease in adulthood by suppressing the natural development of the immune system. Interaction with dirt and germs may actually help to train your immune system!

The most obvious signs of an unhealthy gut are those symptoms which have a clear connection to your digestive system:

- Bloating
- Abdominal pain
- Gas
- Diarrhea
- Constipation
- Acid reflux or heartburn
- Bad breath

Less obvious signs of an unhealthy gut may include symptoms outside of the gut such as:

- Skin conditions (acne, eczema, rosacea)
- Unintentional weight gain or weight loss
- Difficulty losing weight
- Anxiety
- Depression
- Food cravings
- Fatigue
- Vaginosis

Many health conditions, like PCOS and Hashimoto's, are also connected to poor gut health.

Is your gut bacteria causing sugar cravings?

You feed your gut bacteria every time you eat. A diet rich in sugar, fat, and low in fiber leads to overgrowth of the wrong bacteria. These bacteria thrive if you continue to eat this way and they may even direct your behavior in a way that ensures their survival (4). These sugar-loving bacteria influence your food choices and sugar cravings by

- changing your taste receptors to make you prefer sweet flavors;
- releasing happy hormones, like serotonin, to make you feel good after eating certain foods;
- making you feel hungry when you shouldn't be;
- and stimulating your vagus nerve to cause overeating.

Sugar cravings are not the result of poor willpower or discipline. Rather, various factors like dysbiosis, stress, sleep, hormones, and habits all play an influential role in your cravings and eating behavior.

Gut Health and PCOS

By now, you may understand that PCOS involves a chronic state of insulin resistance, high androgen levels, and inflammation. In chapters three through six, we mentioned the factors which influence these three common root causes of PCOS—most notably a poor diet, an unhealthy lifestyle, and stress. Yet, gut health is arguably the most significant factor in the development of PCOS. In fact, some researchers argue that poor gut health is the first trigger in the complex cascade of factors leading to a PCOS diagnosis.

Dysbiosis and PCOS

An imbalance of gut bacteria, or dysbiosis, can cause insulin resistance, hyperandrogenism, and chronic inflammation (1). Some researchers propose a hypothesis called DOGMA (dysbiosis of gut microbiota) which explains a sequence of events causing PCOS:

1. A high-sugar, high-fat, and low-fiber diet causes dysbiosis and damages the tight junctions of the intestinal cells, triggering leaky gut.

2. Leaky gut allows bad bacteria, with lipopolysaccharide (LPS), into the bloodstream which activates the immune system.
3. This activation interferes with insulin signaling, causing insulin resistance.
4. Insulin resistance increases androgens and inflammation, which leads to the common symptoms of PCOS.

If you look at this sequence of events, you may notice that diet and dysbiosis is at the top of the cascade. By addressing your gut health through diet changes and correcting dysbiosis we can disrupt this sequence and potentially reverse your PCOS.

To further study the effect of gut bacteria on PCOS, researchers transplanted feces from healthy women and women with PCOS into two separate groups of mice. Compared to control mice, the mice transplanted with fecal samples from women with PCOS developed insulin resistance, ovarian cysts, and higher levels of testosterone. Researchers also carried out fertility tests and found that the mice given fecal transplants from the PCOS group produced fewer pups than healthy control mice (5).

While we recognize animal studies have some limitations, the collection of research evaluating the gut and PCOS suggest that dysbiosis of your gut bacteria is a main root cause of PCOS. The role of your gut bacteria on the development and progression of PCOS cannot be underestimated!

Side Effects of PCOS Medications

Conventional medications commonly used to manage PCOS symptoms can cause GI symptoms. Metformin is a prescription medication that lowers insulin and fasting blood sugar levels. It is often prescribed to treat insulin resistance in PCOS. While some people see benefits while taking metformin, this drug commonly causes symptoms of GI upset like nausea, diarrhea, bloating, and gas. These side effects may be due to metformin's influence on the gut microbiome, and some studies suggest this drug may also cause dysbiosis. The birth control pill is also commonly prescribed to women with PCOS to manage symptoms of acne, irregular periods, and unwanted hair growth. Unfortunately, many women find that the pill commonly contributes to abdominal bloating among other side effects as well.

The Estrobolome

Your gut microbiome significantly impacts levels of an important hormone called estrogen. During your reproductive years, estrogen is primarily made by your ovaries. A small amount is also made through the conversion of androgens like DHEA or testosterone. Your body is constantly producing estrogen, although the levels should fluctuate throughout your menstrual cycle. After estrogen has its effect on the body, it travels to the liver where it is prepared for elimination through the intestines. Once in the intestines, estrogen is either eliminated or reabsorbed. This is where your gut bacteria come into play.

The estrobolome is the collection of gut bacteria responsible for breaking down and balancing your body's estrogen. When your gut is healthy, these gut bacteria produce normal levels of an enzyme, called beta-glucuronidase. This enzyme turns estrogen into its active form to be reabsorbed by the gut and sent back into the blood. Dysbiosis impairs this process and results in either too much or too little active estrogen. In general, PCOS is a high testosterone and low estrogen condition. Although, we do see PCOS patients with high estrogen levels especially if the patient has long cycles and absent or infrequent ovulation. Nonetheless, women suffering from PCOS have more gut dysbiosis compared to healthy controls, and this likely contributes to an imbalance of estrogen levels (6).

To promote healthy estrogen levels in PCOS, we must treat dysbiosis and promote a bountiful and diverse gut microbiome.

Gut Health and Hashimoto's

Your gut, thyroid gland, and immune system all impact each other in different ways. When one system is disrupted, the others are also affected, and disease can occur. Poor gut health is a major contributing factor to the development of Hashimoto's.

Hashimoto's is an autoimmune disorder in which both genetic predisposition and environmental factors trigger the disease. Studies show that genetics account for about 30 percent of all autoimmune diseases, while the other 70 percent are due to environmental factors like gut dysbiosis, leaky gut, infections, or environmental toxins. Your environment is actually more influential on whether or not you will develop an autoimmune disease than your genetics!

Gut health, and more specifically gut bacteria, play a critical role in normal immune system development. This is because an estimated 70 percent of your immune system resides in your gut through a group of cells called the gut-associated lymphoid tissue (GALT). When gut health is compromised through dysbiosis or leaky gut, your immune system is also affected and autoimmune disease may occur. As we mentioned earlier in this chapter, a variety of factors contribute to dysbiosis of the gut including: diet, alcohol intake, frequent antibiotic use, stress, limited exposure to germs/dirt, and various medications. Dysbiosis eventually impairs the gut lining and causes leaky gut, which allows larger-than-normal food molecules to enter into the intestinal cells. Your immune system mounts an attack on these larger molecules. As more food proteins escape into your bloodstream, your immune system continuously reacts and triggers an inflammatory response. Over time, inflammation disturbs the finely tuned balance of your immune system and it begins to react to non-harmful molecules or even your own cells. This is the basis of autoimmune disease: when your body mistakenly attacks your own organs.

Environmental triggers --> dysbiosis --> leaky gut --> inflammation --> immune system reacts inappropriately --> autoimmune disease

In summary, compromised gut health may cause Hashimoto's by disrupting the immune system. Once the autoimmune disease is present, ongoing gut issues worsen symptoms of Hashimoto's. This may be, in part, due to the role of gut health on the availability and absorption of essential micronutrients for the thyroid gland. When the gut is unhealthy, it cannot as effectively absorb the nutrition you need for optimal health. For example, iron, iodine, and copper are required to make thyroid hormones, selenium and zinc are needed for converting T4 into the active T3 hormone, and vitamin D is essential for controlling the immune system response (7). Individuals with Hashimoto's are often deficient in these nutrients.

Constipation and Hypothyroidism

In hypothyroidism, the movement of food through the GI tract is slowed, which is why many individuals with this condition complain of constipation. Unfortunately, a slower GI motility increases the risk of bacterial overgrowth (dysbiosis) and studies have found over half of patients with hypothyroidism to have bacterial overgrowth (8). This begs the question: does hypothyroidism cause dysbiosis, or does dysbiosis cause hypothyroidism? While there may be a bidirectional relationship, bacterial overgrowth is also seen in hyperthyroidism (an "overactive" thyroid), which suggests that the overgrowth causes thyroid disease and not the other way around.

Testing for Gut Health

Depending on your individual case, there are a few functional lab tests your doctor may order to gather further information. Keep in mind, these tests are not generally covered by insurance, and conventional practitioners usually do not order them. These tests are best ordered by a functional medicine provider who knows how to interpret them and form interventions based on your results.

Breath Testing

A breath test is used to diagnose a condition called small intestinal bacterial overgrowth (SIBO). Most of your gut bacteria are supposed to live in your colon. When too many bacteria colonize the small intestine, you can experience unpleasant symptoms, like acne, bloating, and diarrhea or constipation. SIBO is also connected to higher levels of inflammation, and conditions like leaky gut and hypothyroidism.

In a SIBO breath test, you drink a specific syrup and provide breath samples at various time intervals. The bacteria in your small intestine feed on the syrup and produce hydrogen and/or methane gas. If the levels of gas are higher than the provided threshold, this may indicate a SIBO diagnosis.

Stool Testing

A stool test is helpful when looking at the health of the colon. We use functional stool tests with our patients at Root Functional Medicine. For this test, our patients collect an at-home stool sample and ship it to the laboratory with the provided mailing kit. The stool test looks for gut pathogens (i.e. bad bugs), dysbiosis, parasites, and other intestinal health markers like calprotectin (inflammation), IgA (immune function), and beta-glucuronidase (estrogen metabolism).

Both breath and stool testing allow functional medicine practitioners to form an individualized treatment plan based on what is happening in your own gut.

Restoring Gut Health

As you can imagine, restoring gut health can be a complex process best carried out with an experienced doctor. However, you will learn about the gut health protocol we use at Root in our 3 month plan discussed in this book. Thankfully, there are many things you can personally do to improve the health of your gut. While it may seem overwhelming at first, keep in mind that you can actually alter the composition of your gut bacteria in as little as five days!

Reduce gut disruptors

An important first step in restoring gut health is elimination of factors that are harmful to the gut. Diet arguably has the largest impact on your gut health because these foods come into contact with your gut bacteria multiple times per day. Added sugar disrupts your gut bacteria by feeding the harmful bugs and starving the good bugs.

The largest sources of added sugar in the standard American diet are sugar-sweetened beverages and desserts or sweet snacks. This is a great place to start. Aim to reduce or eliminate regular intake of these items. Examples of sugar-sweetened beverages include sweetened coffee, soda, juice, and sweet tea. Many beverages contain added sugar even if they are marketed as "healthy" options. Get into the habit of briefly checking the ingredient label to look for these sneaky sources of sugar. New labeling requirements make this process easier by including a separate line on the nutrition facts label to clearly show how many grams of added sugar are in each serving of the product. Lower is better!

Eat a fiber-rich diet

While we work to starve the bad bugs by reducing added sugar, we want to simultaneously feed the good bugs. This is where fiber comes into play. Fiber is the preferred source of fuel for your beneficial gut bacteria. Eating fiber-rich foods with our meals and snacks ensures the survival and growth of good gut bacteria which then provide benefits like reduced inflammation, healthy estrogen metabolism, regular bowel movements, and more. You should aim to eat at least 25 grams of fiber per day. If you have trouble tolerating this much fiber, consider working with your doctor to obtain a test for SIBO as discussed above.

Some high fiber foods include

- **Non-starchy vegetables:** broccoli, Brussels sprouts, cauliflower, carrot
- **Starchy vegetables:** potato, sweet potato, winter squash
- **Fruit:** apple, banana, blueberries, raspberries, pear, orange
- **Grains:** quinoa, oats, brown rice
- **Legumes, nuts, and seeds:** green peas, lentils, black beans, chia seeds, almonds, pistachios

Include a variety of foods

To cultivate a diverse gut microbiome, you need to eat a colorful and diverse diet. The standard "chicken, broccoli, and rice" meal, while still healthy if balanced protein, fat, and fiber, offers little for your gut bacteria when no other foods are included in your regular meal roundup. Likewise, popular diets like low-carb or ketogenic diets contain too little fiber and restrict many of the above foods which are required for optimal gut health. These diets may initially promote weight loss and blood sugar balance, however, their lower fiber and restrictive nature makes it a poor diet option for gut diversity.

Following the Protein + Fat + Carbohydrate and Root Plate methods described in earlier chapters and in chapter eight encourages balanced and diverse meals for optimal gut health.

Get dirty

Live a lifestyle that supports microbial diversity. Spend time in nature, play with your pets, work in your garden, and enjoy the outdoors whenever possible! These lifestyle factors expose you to other diverse bugs. Avoid overusing antibacterial soaps and cleaning products that may also kill the unharmful or beneficial bacteria in your environment.

Key Takeaways

- Dysbiosis of the gut is a major root cause of both PCOS and Hashimoto's by causing leaky gut and triggering inflammation.

- Treating dysbiosis in PCOS and Hashimoto's can improve insulin resistance and thereby reduce androgens, inflammation, and many related symptoms.
- You can start restoring gut health by reducing added sugar, eating a diverse, fiber-rich diet, and exposing yourself to other beneficial bacteria in nature.

8

Food First Plan

PCOS and Hashimoto's are complex conditions and, as you've learned, they have multiple root causes. At first, it may seem overwhelming. Where do you even begin? Instead of chasing symptoms with strict diets or temporary treatments, we will teach you how to address the root cause of your PCOS and/or Hashimoto's with food, lifestyle, and targeted supplementation. These three pillars address all possible root causes and many interventions even overlap to address more than one root cause. In this chapter, we will provide our tried and true 3-month plan to treat PCOS and Hashimoto's and achieve hormonal harmony.

Before we get started, let's briefly review the five root causes of PCOS and Hashimoto's we discussed in the first half of the book. While we know it's tempting to skip ahead, we encourage you to refresh your memory of this important information so you understand "the why" behind our recommendations.

Root Cause #1: Insulin Resistance

Insulin resistance occurs when your cells do not respond properly to insulin leading to high levels of sugar and insulin in your blood. Insulin resistance drives inflammation which worsens symptoms of both PCOS and Hashimoto's. Insulin resistance also causes an increase in androgen levels, like testosterone. Up to 70 percent of women with PCOS have some degree of insulin resistance as one of their root causes.

Root Cause #2: Testosterone

Androgens are commonly referred to as "male" hormones but are produced by women as well. When your body produces too many androgens, as seen in PCOS and some cases of Hashimoto's, you may experience acne, unwanted hair growth or hair loss, and irregular periods.

Root Cause #3: Adrenal Health

HPA axis dysfunction is the third root cause of PCOS and Hashimoto's thyroid disease. This is when your body produces too many stress hormones, like cortisol or DHEA-S. High cortisol levels may cause PCOS by increasing blood sugar levels, worsening insulin resistance, and triggering weight gain. High cortisol levels also lower active thyroid hormone and increase reverse T3, which can slow metabolism and worsen hypothyroidism.

Root Cause #4: Mitochondrial Health

Mitochondrial dysfunction is the fourth root cause of both PCOS and Hashimoto's. Oxidative stress (from diet, lifestyle, and/or environmental toxins) damages the mitochondria and makes them less efficient at producing energy. Damaged mitochondria may then lead to several characteristics of PCOS and Hashimoto's like insulin resistance, period irregularities or infertility, and worsening hypothyroidism.

Root Cause #5: Gut Health

Dysbiosis of the gut is arguably the most influential root cause of both PCOS and Hashimoto's because it can be the impetus of all other root causes. While we will address interventions for gut health in this chapter with the foods you eat, we've also dedicated the entirety of chapter nine to treating gut imbalances as well. Dysbiosis creates the chronic low grade inflammation that is a hallmark root cause of both PCOS and Hashimoto's.

Before You Get Started

You may have started implementing some of the strategies we discussed in the first half of the book to address the multiple root causes of PCOS and Hashimoto's. If so, wonderful! If not, don't worry! We will walk you through everything you need to know.

Labs

In addition to receiving our 3-month plan, our 1:1 members also undergo individualized lab testing that helps us modify treatments to their specific needs. While this is a major part of functional medicine, you do not need these labs to see improvements or follow our 3-month plan outlined in the book. However, labs are a great way to not only tailor interventions, but also track progress.

If you would like to obtain baseline labs, you may be able to request these from your primary care physician. However, please check with your insurance company before assuming any coverage. Alternatively, there are some companies which allow you to select and purchase your lab tests online without insurance or a prescription, like anylabtestnow.com, ultalabtests.com, and directlabs.com. Furthermore, there are some tests we order in our clinic that are not covered by insurance and require a functional medicine practitioner who knows how to interpret the results and develop appropriate interventions. While we will discuss these tests throughout the next few chapters, we do not recommend ordering them yourself without professional guidance.

Here are the baseline labs we encourage you to request from your primary care physician:

- Hemoglobin a1c
- Fasting insulin
- Fasting blood glucose
- HS-CRP
- Testosterone

- DHEA-S
- TSH
- Free T4
- Free T3
- Thyroid Peroxidase Antibodies (TPO Ab)

It is important to work with your doctor to interpret the results of these labs. But remember, these labs are not required to follow our 3-month plan.

Evaluate Your Relationship with Food

Your overall diet—as in the foods you eat—is a powerful tool to find healing in many different areas of PCOS and Hashimoto's. However, we also recognize diet culture particularly targets women who suffer from ongoing health conditions. Especially in functional medicine, people often feel like they need to restrict or eliminate multiple food groups to find success. We find that individuals may also feel guilty, ashamed, or embarrassed of their past or present food choices. They may also feel preoccupied with food and cycle through periods of restriction followed by binging. If any of this resonates with you, please take a moment to read and reflect on these main points before moving forward with the 3-month plan:

- Food does not have any moral value and is not inherently "good" or "bad."
- Shift your focus from outward food rules to how different foods make you feel physically, emotionally, and mentally. A food/mood journal is a great way to briefly note the foods you are eating and how they make you feel.
- You don't have to eat a perfect diet to achieve results. Progress and consistency, not perfection, is what matters.
- It is important to find ways to comfort and resolve your emotions without using food.

Forming a healthy relationship with food takes conscious effort, but it is possible! While we pride ourselves in taking a sustainable and realistic approach to nutrition, please talk with your doctor before starting any new program, especially if you previously or currently suffer from an eating disorder.

Initial Symptom Survey

A symptom survey is a document used to evaluate your symptoms and track progress or pinpoint areas of focus. We like our members to take these surveys before starting their treatment plan, after one month of changes, and after about three months. You will be amazed at how simple changes will reduce multiple symptoms in just weeks!

Take a few minutes now to fill out your initial symptom survey. You can find a sample symptom survey in the appendix of this book.

Pantry and Freezer Staples

Consider stocking your pantry and freezer with nutritious staples. Keeping these food items on hand makes it easier to add nutrient-dense foods to your meals and snacks each day.

Fats:

- Olive oil
- Avocado oil
- Coconut oil
- Sesame oil
- Pumpkin seeds
- Chia seeds
- Flaxseeds
- Hemp seeds
- Sunflower seeds
- Almond flour

- Nut/seed butters (peanut, almond, sunflower)

Tip: Keep nuts and seeds in the refrigerator or freezer if you don't think you will use them right away or if you purchase them in bulk.

Dried goods/spices:

- Canned beans (2-3 types)
- Canned fish (salmon, tuna, sardines)
- Rolled oats (gluten free if needed)
- Spices (at minimum):
  - Salt
  - Pepper
  - Cinnamon
  - Garlic powder
  - Oregano
  - Parsley
  - Italian seasoning
  - Cumin
  - Dill
  - Rosemary
  - Thyme
  - Paprika
- Coconut aminos
- Store-bought vegetable broth or bone broth
- Rice
- Quinoa
- Collagen peptides or single ingredient protein powders such as pea protein, flaxseed protein, or pumpkin seed protein

Freezer:

- Frozen vegetables to heat for easy sides
- Frozen berries
- Frozen fish, poultry, and other meats

Month One

The goal of our Root Protocol is to treat the five root causes, eliminate your related symptoms, and help you achieve hormonal harmony with sustainable changes. The first month of our 3-month plan includes a diet rehaul with our Hormone Balancing Meal Plan and targeted supplementation.

In general, during this first month you will

- consume a variety of colorful vegetables and fruit;
- balance meals and snacks with protein, healthy fat, and carbo-hydrates (fiber);
- cook the majority of meals from home;
- remove added sugar and refined carbohydrates;
- implement an overnight 12-hour fast;
- start the recommended supplements.

To begin, let's review your diet rehaul using our Hormone Balancing Meal Plan.

The Hormone Balancing Meal Plan

PFC Balance

The Root Plate Method for PFC balance is the first essential tool in our meal plan. PFC is a simple formula that ensures you have protein, fat, and fiber-rich carbohydrates on each plate. Each of these macronutrients play a vital role in PCOS and Hashimoto's, which is why we need a proper balance of all three.

The Root Plate™

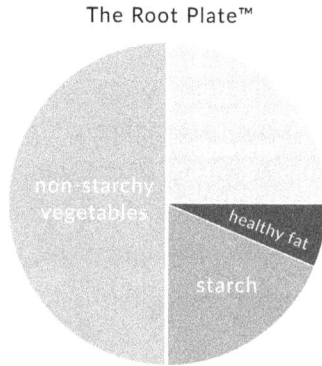

Protein

Protein is essential for human health and offers many benefits for PCOS and Hashimoto's like

- slowing digestion and preventing blood sugar spikes;
- increasing satiety after a meal (this can reduce sugar cravings too);
- offering essential nutrients like zinc, iron, vitamin B6, and vitamin B12.

Rich sources of protein include: beef, pork, seafood, poultry, and eggs. Some plants also contain protein like tofu and edamame. Though legumes, lentils, and beans contain some protein, they also contain mostly carbohydrates so we put these in the starch category of the plate when considering balancing blood sugars.

When choosing animal protein, prioritize high-quality sources from grass-fed, pasture-raised, or wild-caught animals. Compared to grain-fed animals, grass-fed meats are higher in healthy omega-3 fats, vitamin A, and vitamin E. We recognize that these protein options are usually more expensive than grain-fed alternatives. Shop the sale ads when possible, and check your local big box store as they often sell these options for a lower price per pound than traditional grocery stores. Alternatively, you can also check with local farmers and ranchers in your area to discuss options for purchasing locally raised meat.

It's also important to note that high quality animal protein at only the size of your palm will get you to 20-30 grams of protein. As we will discuss later in this chapter, protein should only fill about ¼ of your plate. When this method is implemented, many people find that they can stretch their dollar further while purchasing higher quality meat.

Fat

Fat is another macronutrient needed to make hormones, balance blood sugar levels, and help absorb essential vitamins. Including healthy fats in your diet may also help to reduce inflammation and aid weight loss. Try to prioritize including healthier fats into your meals, such as those found in olive oil, avocados, coconut oil, nuts, seeds, and fatty fish.

Carbohydrates

Carbohydrates can have a bad reputation these days, and low-carb or ketogenic diets have skyrocketed in popularity. However, we find that these diets are difficult to maintain, trigger sugar cravings, and often do not provide enough calories. A diet too low in calories may actually worsen your menstrual cycle and hypothyroidism!

Rather than avoiding carbohydrates altogether, focus on prioritizing foods rich in *complex* carbohydrates instead. Complex carbohydrates digest slowly, keep you fuller for longer, and prevent blood sugar spikes. These food sources also offer essential b-complex vitamins and nourishing fiber to feed your healthy gut bacteria. We recommend gradually increasing fiber intake to a goal of 25 to 35 grams per day. The end goal is to be closer to 35 grams of fiber.

There are four main types of foods that contain complex carbohydrates:

- Fruit
- Starchy vegetables
- Whole grains
- Non-starchy vegetables

Refer to appendix PCOS Thyroid Recipes for recipes that fit the Root Plate.

The Root Plate

The Root Plate is a great way to visualize PFC Balance without having to measure out portions or count calories. With this method, a quarter of your plate contains a protein source, the other quarter contains a source of complex carbohydrates, and half of your plate is full of non-starchy vegetables. We also recommend a serving of healthy fats as well, since fat is foundational in making sex hormones, balancing blood sugar, and keeping you satisfied after a meal.

Phytonutrients

Phytonutrients are compounds made by plants that provide desirable health benefits to humans. It is the phytonutrients that give plant-based foods their unique color! For example, lycopene and beta-carotene are phytochemicals found in red foods, like tomatoes. Anthocyanins are found in blue and purple foods, like berries, and quercetin is found in brown and white foods, like quinoa, onions, and beans.

Phytonutrients are crucial for women with PCOS and Hashimoto's because they boost antioxidant levels in the body and provide anti-inflammatory benefits. Since each color generally represents a different type of phytonutrient, aim to make each plate as colorful as possible to ensure that you are consuming a wide variety of these antioxidants.

Intermittent Fasting

Intermittent fasting is the term used to describe various fasting patterns in which you purposefully fast for a specified amount of time. For the next three months, we recommend implementing a 12-hour overnight fast (water is fine) at least five days of the week. This means if you stopped eating at 7 p.m, you would eat breakfast the next day around 7 a.m if you are awake and hungry at that time. The main benefits of intermittent fasting found in research so far include fat loss, improvements in fasting blood sugar, and reduced insulin resistance (1, 2). Intermittent fasting may also reduce levels of inflammation within the body (3). However, please do not try to fast for longer periods of time during these three months. Long periods of fasting may lead to disordered eating behaviors, a diet too low in calories, and higher cortisol levels.

Pro tip: If you are feeling extremely hungry between 8-10 p.m., consider examining the following: 1) Was my plate PFC balanced? Did I eat enough veggies, protein, and fat? 2) Am I eating dinner too early? Perhaps shifting dinner from 5 p.m. to 6:30 p.m. and planning on having a PFC balanced snack at 3-4 p.m. would serve you better. On the days you choose to eat something at night, having a small handful of nuts can be helpful to reduce hunger and stomach growling and give you adequate protein & fat to keep blood sugar balanced while you sleep.

Hormone Balancing Meal Plan

The cornerstones of this meal plan include PFC balance using the Root Plate in addition to:

- 25 to 35 grams of dietary fiber per day for blood sugar balance and proper elimination of toxins and hormones
- Aim for 20-30 grams of protein at breakfast, lunch, and dinner
- Fish 2 to 3 times per week for anti-inflammatory omega-3, selenium, and iodine
- At least one serving of nuts and seeds daily for zinc, magnesium, and omega-3
- Frequent consumption of cruciferous vegetables to promote estrogen balance
- Beans 2 to 3 times per week for antioxidants and fiber
- Eggs at least twice per week for choline and fertility support
- Daily spearmint or green tea for anti-androgenic properties

See appendix for recipes and food inspiration.

Foods to Limit in Month One

Our Hormone Balancing Meal Plan focuses on nutrient density and adding more color and variety into your meals and snacks as well as balancing your plate for blood sugar balance. Our goal is to address your root causes of PCOS and Hashimoto's and eliminate your symptoms with the least restrictive diet possible. Therefore, in this first month, we will not ask you to remove very many foods from your diet. Nonetheless, we do recommend removing a few types of foods in this first month that may, when eaten in excess, worsen PCOS and Hashimoto's.

Added Sugar

There are some naturally occurring sugars—like those found in fruit —and there are sugars which manufacturers add to food products—appropriately named "added sugar." We recommend removing all sources of added sugar throughout the 3-month plan. Consuming too much added sugar can worsen insulin resistance, raise androgen levels, cause gut dysbiosis, and worsen inflammation.

While our program does not require counting calories or excessive label reading, we encourage awareness of the nutrition facts label to help guide food choices, when applicable.

Thankfully, new changes to the nutrition facts label clearly show the amount of added sugar in a packaged food. "Total sugars" include sugars naturally present in the food or beverage PLUS any added sugars in the product. While this line is important, you should pay more attention to the next line. The "added sugars" line includes sugars that are added during food processing. Manufacturers may add ingredients like dextrose, table sugar, syrups, honey, or concentrated fruit juice.

The biggest sources of added sugars in the American diet are sugar-sweetened beverages, baked goods, desserts, and other sweets. Focus on reducing or eliminating these main sources first, and then begin to swap out hidden sources of added sugars, like yogurt, granola bars, packaged oatmeal, condiments, and "original" flavored nut or oat milks. When cutting out sources of added sugar, make sure to check the ingredient list to ensure that there are no artificial sweeteners in the product either.

When you focus on PFC balance and eating whole foods, added sugars and artificial sweeteners will be automatically reduced.

The Role of Fruit in Your Meal Plan

Fruit is often villainized in PCOS and Hashimoto's because of its carbohydrate content. However, fruit is a type of complex carbohydrate that offers many benefits to a hormone balancing meal plan. Whole fruit offers fiber, anti-inflammatory phytonutrients, and essential nutrients like vitamin C. Not to mention, fruit is delicious and enjoyable! You will notice that we include various sources of fruit in our recipes, especially berries, as they are particularly rich in antioxidants and do not spike blood sugar levels as much as other fruits or fruit juices without fiber. Additionally, we always pair fruit with a protein or fat source, like nuts and seeds. This ensures blood sugar stability and promotes satiety. Avoid fruit sources that may have added sugar, like fruit juice or canned fruit.

Artificial Sweeteners

Artificial sweeteners, also known as zero-calorie sweeteners, are often disguised in products labeled as "sugar-free." However, these sweeteners can be up to 20,000 times sweeter than regular sugar and overstimulate your taste receptors. Unfortunately, this may actually reduce your taste preferences for less sweet, more complex flavors (like fruit and vegetables). Artificial sweeteners also disrupt gut health by negatively influencing the balance of your gut bacteria. For these reasons, we recommend avoiding artificial sweeteners during your 3-month plan as well. Artificial sugars are NOT included in the "added sugars" line on the nutrition facts label. Food manufacturers are only required to list these zero-calorie sweeteners among the ingredients.

Look for these common artificial sweeteners in the ingredient line:

- aspartame
- acesulfame potassium
- neotame
- saccharin
- sucralose
- stevia
- sugar alcohols (erythritol, mannitol, xylitol, sorbitol)

If a product is advertised as "sugar-free", double check for hints of these artificial sweeteners.

Caffeine & Alcohol

Don't worry, we won't make you give up coffee! However, in excess, caffeine can worsen HPA dysfunction and disrupt healthy sleep patterns. We recommend reducing caffeine intake to 12 fluid ounces or less per day. Please also limit your caffeine intake to before 12 noon, if possible. Caffeine intake later in the day disrupts your sleep cycle and normal cortisol patterns. If you struggle to make it through the day without an afternoon cup of coffee, this is a sure sign that you need to start cutting back now! While some individuals find it easier to slowly wean themselves off of caffeine, others may prefer to do it "cold turkey." Keep in mind, you may get a caffeine-withdrawal headache if you choose to go cold turkey. If desired, you can swap out your afternoon caffeine source with alternative beverage choices like filtered or sparkling water, unsweetened coconut water, green or herbal tea (especially spearmint tea which has PCOS/thyroid benefits), or decaf coffee.

We also recommend limiting alcohol to less than two drinks per week or eliminating it completely during this 3-month period. Better drink choices if you do choose to have them are wine because it does contain antioxidants, or keeping it simple with plain soda water, 1oz of vodka and a splash of citrus. Remember 5 oz is considered one glass and each bottle is technically 5 glasses of wine. There are also several new mocktail beverages on the market you could drink instead of an alcoholic beverage. One of our favorites is hop water, which is also gluten free.

Keep in mind that many alcoholic beverages, coffee creamers, and lattes contain a significant amount of added sugar!

Pro tip: Coffee shops typically add 3 pumps of syrup (at about 5 grams of sugar per pump) to a small latte. If you would like to still enjoy an occasional latte, ask them to put just 1 pump of syrup in your latte (you will save 10 grams of sugar) and pair your drink with a handful of nuts & seeds to help with blood sugar stabilization. If you want to try your latte syrup-free (recommended), try shaking on some cinnamon, pumpkin spice, or ginger on top of your drink for subtle/natural sweetness.

Core Supplements for Month One

We prioritize food first in all of our treatment plans. However, there is also a place for targeted supplements when treating PCOS and

Hashimoto's. In this first month, we recommend starting a few core supplements that are proven to treat the various root causes of PCOS and Hashimoto's. While you are free to purchase these supplements elsewhere, we do offer our PCOS Core Supplement Bundle on our website at rootfunctionalmedicine.com/shop-root.

Inositol

Inositol is one of the best supplements for PCOS and Hashimoto's due to its ability to reduce insulin resistance by normalizing blood sugar and insulin levels (4). Inositol is also useful in lowering TSH and thyroid antibody levels (5, 6).

By improving insulin resistance with inositol, you may experience more regular menstrual cycles, enhanced fertility, and lower testosterone levels. In fact, one study found that myo-inositol was more effective in restoring ovulation than metformin, a drug commonly used to treat insulin resistance in PCOS (7).

The two main types of inositol are called myo-inositol and D-chiro-inositol. Taking a 40:1 combination of myo- and D-chiro-inositol mimics the ratio of these molecules naturally found in the body. We recommend taking 2 grams of inositol twice daily (morning and night).

N-Acetyl Cysteine (NAC)

NAC is a powerful antioxidant that reduces inflammation and oxidative stress in the body. Oxidative stress occurs when you have too many free radicals and/or too little antioxidants. Women with PCOS and Hashimoto's tend to have higher levels of inflammation and oxidative stress, which is why NAC is another key supplement in our 3-month plan.

By lowering inflammation and oxidative stress, studies show NAC can

- lower testosterone levels (8);
- improve insulin resistance and reduce fasting insulin (9);
- boost fertility by optimizing ovulation and improving cervical mucus quality (10).

NAC is a safe and well-tolerated supplement. We recommend taking around 900-1800 mg of NAC every day.

Omega-3

Omega-3 is a healthy fatty acid that can lower inflammation, increase antioxidant levels, and improve energy production in the mitochondria (11). Fish oil is a specific type of omega-3 fat derived from oily fish like salmon, herring, and anchovies. Fish oil also has powerful anti-inflammatory benefits and may improve insulin resistance and lower cholesterol numbers in women with PCOS (12).

Fish oil, or omega-3 supplements, should contain the two key omega-3 fats derived from fish: EPA and DHA. In addition to eating fish 1 - 2 times per week, we recommend taking around 1,000 mg of total fish oil (EPA + DHA) per day.

Magnesium

Magnesium is involved in over 300 reactions in the body, many of which affect hormone balance and signaling. Unfortunately, over two-thirds of Americans fail to meet the daily magnesium requirements with their diet. Individuals with PCOS are particularly more likely to under consume magnesium-rich foods and have a greater likelihood of having lower magnesium levels. Adequate magnesium intake is essential for promoting healthy blood sugar and insulin levels in addition to reducing inflammation(13). Magnesium also has a calming effect and promotes restful sleep, which helps to balance cortisol levels and improve adrenal health.

Magnesium supplements are available in a variety of forms, including magnesium oxide, citrate, or bisglycinate. Magnesium oxide is not well absorbed and may cause diarrhea or GI upset. Magnesium citrate, however, is much better tolerated and has a very gentle laxative effect which may help if you also suffer from constipation. Magnesium bisglycinate is the most universal form that is well absorbed and tolerated with minimal GI effects. We recommend taking 200 mg of magnesium citrate or bisglycinate every day.

Optional Supplements

Our Root PCOS Supplement Bundle including Inositol, NAC, Magnesium, and Omega 3s is highly recommended and effective for our patients with PCOS and Hashimoto's. However, there are a few other optional supplements which may be helpful depending on your circumstances.

Vitamin D

Up to 85 percent of women with PCOS have a vitamin D deficiency. Similarly, vitamin D deficiency is common in Hashimoto's thyroid disease and treating this deficiency may even slow down the development of hypothyroidism.

Most labs suggest that normal vitamin D levels are 30 ng/mL or higher and deficiency is 20 ng/mL or lower. However, a "normal level" does not necessarily mean optimal. For our patients, we aim for vitamin D levels around 50 ng/mL for best outcomes.

Since vitamin D is not commonly found in the foods we eat, we must rely on adequate sunshine or supplementation. Supplementing with vitamin D may improve insulin resistance, lower inflammation, and help to normalize your menstrual cycle (13). Vitamin D supplements should be personalized based on your own lab results. For example, if your vitamin D levels are adequate (50 ng/mL), a maintenance dose of about 2,000 units per day may be most appropriate depending on where you live and the time of the year. However, you may require higher doses (5,000 units per day) if your blood levels indicate a vitamin D inadequacy or deficiency. If you are severely deficient, you may require a short term prescription for a megadose of vitamin D.

We order vitamin D labs on all of our 1:1 patients in our practice because of the widespread deficiency in the PCOS and Hashimoto's population. If required, your vitamin D supplement should also contain vitamin K2, which helps direct calcium and vitamin D to your bones where it can be used and stored. We also offer a vitamin D/K2 supplement containing 5,000 units of vitamin D on our online root shop at rootfunctionalmedicine.com/shop-root. If you are curious about your vitamin D levels, you can request this lab from your primary care doctor.

B-Complex Vitamin

A general B-complex vitamin is another optional supplement you may consider taking. Medications often prescribed for PCOS (like birth control and metformin) can deplete your body of many important B vitamins. Vitamin B6, folate, and vitamin B12 are particularly important in optimizing hormonal balance. These three B-vitamins help to lower inflammation by breaking down an amino acid, called homocysteine, which is commonly elevated in women with PCOS. Lowering homocysteine may reduce your risk factors for heart disease and other reproductive symptoms. Choose a B-complex vitamin that contains the methylated forms of folate and vitamin B12. These methylated forms (named methylfolate and methylcobalamin, respectively) are the active version of these vitamins and more effectively used by the body. If you are trying to conceive, taking metformin or the birth control pill, or recently off the pill, we would encourage you to add a B-complex vitamin to your regimen as well.

Zinc

Zinc is an essential mineral found primarily in animal products, nuts, seeds, and beans. Zinc acts as an antioxidant and has proven benefits for treating insulin resistance by lowering blood sugar and insulin levels, treating unwanted hair loss or acne (symptoms of high androgens), and supporting thyroid health (14, 15). In fact, zinc is required to convert T4 thyroid hormone into the active T3 version for your body to use.

If you suffer from hair loss, unwanted hair growth, or acne, you may want to add zinc to your supplement regimen. We recommend taking around 15 to 30 mg of zinc per day.

Summary of Month One

Month one of our 3-month program is a diet rehaul using our Hormone Balancing Meal Plan intended to address all five root causes of PCOS and Hashimoto's: insulin resistance, testosterone, adrenal health, mitochondrial dysfunction, and gut health. We are not looking for perfection during this time, so if you fall off the program for a day or two, do not give up! Changing your food habits takes time, repetition, and a lot of grace. That being said, we encourage you to take this month seriously. These next thirty days are going to pass whether you stick to the program or not. At the end of the month, wouldn't you rather look back and feel gratitude for how much you have accomplished? While this program is specifically tailored to individuals with PCOS and Hashimoto's, any person can benefit from the food recommendations in this plan. If needed, get your spouse, partner, family member, or friend to join you for increased accountability and motivation!

As a reminder, during this month you will

- consume a variety of colorful vegetables and fruit;
- balance meals and snacks with protein, healthy fat, and carbohydrates (fiber);

- cook the majority of meals from home;
- remove added sugar and refined carbohydrates;
- implement an overnight 12-hour fast;
- start the recommended supplements (inositol, NAC, omega-3, and magnesium).

Depending on your circumstances, you may also want to start taking vitamin D, a B-complex vitamin, and/or supplemental zinc.

Month Two

You made it through the first month, congratulations! Even if month one did not go as smoothly as you may have hoped, remember that we are aiming for progress over perfection. Did you eat more colorful and fresh foods than before the program? Did you reduce your added sugar intake at all? Did you cook more meals from home? If you answered yes to any of these questions, then you are already making great progress! The next step is to re-take your symptom survey.

Compare your initial symptom survey to your follow-up survey and answer the next few questions to reflect on your progress. Did your grand total score decrease? Did your score decrease in certain categories but remain the same or increase in other categories? Reflecting back on the past month, how consistent were you with the recommended meal plan and supplements?

If you followed the food and supplement plan with at least 75 percent consistency and are still experiencing symptoms, you may require a few more tweaks to your food plan for month two (we will discuss these below). If you were less than 75 percent consistent, you may consider restarting month one. There is no shame in this decision! In fact, it is extremely important that you build a strong foundation with the month one recommendations rather than half-heartedly going through the motions without true intention. Lastly, if you are satisfied with your improvement in symptoms after month one, you may not need to restrict your diet any further! In this case, continue with the food plan and recommended supplements from month one throughout the remainder of the program. Either way, keep in mind that it may take three months or longer to see significant changes and symptom relief. True healing takes time! Do not let your motivation waver or give in to an unproven quick fix. In this second month, we recommend continuing all interventions from month one.

Depending on the above circumstances, during this second month, you will trial a complete elimination of gluten, dairy, soy, and corn.

Gluten

Gluten is the name for a group of proteins found in grains like wheat, barley, and rye. Gluten provides texture, retains moisture, and promotes elasticity to bread and other baked goods.

Everyday foods that commonly contain gluten include:

- Pasta
- Bread
- Crackers
- Cookies
- Pastries
- Cakes or Pies
- Cereal
- Beer

Because of its unique properties, gluten is also used as an additive in some processed foods like gravy, condiments, soup, and lunchmeat.

There are two main types of gluten-related disorders: celiac disease and non-celiac gluten sensitivity. Celiac disease is a serious autoimmune condition in which a person's immune system mistakenly attacks the lining of their small intestine after eating gluten-containing foods. The only treatment for celiac disease is a strict and lifelong gluten-free diet.

An estimated one percent of the general population has celiac disease. Although, the prevalence of celiac disease is higher (up to five percent) in people with Hashimoto's thyroid autoimmunity (16, 17). For this reason, we often screen our members with Hashimoto's for celiac disease. Your doctor can screen for celiac disease with a blood test to look for antibodies called anti-tissue transglutaminase (tTGA). However, this screen must be done before you eliminate gluten from your diet. Testing for celiac disease after a few days of following a gluten-free diet may result in a false negative test result.

The second type of gluten-related disorder is gluten sensitivity. This is a condition in which a person experiences a variety of symptoms after eating gluten-containing foods, but does not have celiac disease or a wheat allergy. Symptoms of gluten sensitivity vary and may include gastrointestinal upset, brain fog, anxiety, headaches, or skin disturbances. Gluten sensitivity is thought to affect up to 13 percent of the general population and may be more prevalent in women than men. Currently, there is no universally agreed upon method to diagnose gluten sensitivity.

Why We Recommend Eliminating Gluten in Month Two

Currently, there are no research studies to support a blanket gluten-free diet recommendation for all women with PCOS. However, some studies have shown benefits for using a gluten-free diet with Hashimoto's in reducing thyroid antibody levels (18, 19).

Nonetheless, many of our patients with PCOS and Hashimoto's report feeling better on a gluten-free diet. This could be due to the fact that most gluten-containing foods in the American diet are also higher in refined carbohydrates and/or added sugar. However, it may be due to gluten sensitivity. While gluten sensitivity does not cause PCOS or Hashimoto's, it is often a symptom of an underlying imbalance, like poor gut health and inflammation.

We recommend eliminating gluten completely during month two, especially if you reported lingering symptoms on your follow-up symptom survey after month one. It's important to note that many gluten-free food items have poor nutritional value and a lot of added sugar. Instead of swapping out your gluten-containing foods for processed gluten-free alternatives, focus on eating more whole and unprocessed foods that are naturally free of gluten like fruits, vegetables, nuts, seeds, lean protein, and gluten-free whole grains (i.e. brown rice or quinoa).

Dairy

Like gluten, there are limited published studies to support a blanket recommendation of a dairy-free diet for all individuals with PCOS and Hashimoto's. Some studies show an increased frequency of acne in individuals consuming more skim or low-fat milk. Low-fat dairy foods have also been associated with high androgen levels, which may explain why these foods are also linked to worsening acne. Furthermore, a large prospective study found that high intake of low-fat dairy products may increase a woman's risk of ovulation-related infertility, while high-fat dairy foods may decrease the risk of this condition (20). PCOS is the most common cause of ovulation-related infertility.

The case for a dairy-free diet is nuanced and highly individualized. Similar to gluten, we find that many patients have a dairy sensitivity, lactose intolerance, or simply feel better on a dairy-free diet. In fact, lactose intolerance is fairly common in Hashimoto's, with one small study reporting lactose intolerance in 75 percent of their test subjects. This same study found that lactose restriction significantly decreased TSH levels in patients with Hashimoto's (21). The only way to evaluate your body's reaction to dairy is to temporarily eliminate it from your diet, which is why we include this recommendation in month two of our three month plan.

If you choose to keep dairy into your diet, choose organic, pasture-raised, and whole-fat dairy products. Alternatively, if you choose to trial a dairy elimination, keep in mind that some dairy-free products contain high amounts of added sugar or artificial sweeteners. Choose unsweetened nut, oat, or coconut milk products, and nutritional yeast or a DIY cashew sauce for cheese alternatives in recipes.

Soy

Soy comes from a soybean plant with pods that produce a type of legume. Like other legumes, soy is a nutrient-dense source of plant protein. In fact, one cup of shelled edamame (immature soybeans) contains 19 grams of protein and 8 grams of fiber! Soybeans are also rich in important nutrients like iron, magnesium, folate, and vitamin K.

Whole food sources of soy include:

- Soybeans
- Edamame
- Tofu
- Soy milk
- Tempeh
- Miso
- Natto

However, most Americans consume soy in the form of soy-based additives which manufacturers add to packaged food products like soybean oil, soy lecithin, and soy protein isolate. You may find these ingredients in protein powder/shakes, veggie burgers, and other meat substitutes. These sources of soy are less healthy because the natural nutrients found in soy are stripped and processed away.

Despite what you may think, soy does have some proven benefits for women with PCOS. First of all, soy intake may improve metabolic health by lowering LDL cholesterol, triglycerides, and free insulin levels. Thanks in part to its favorable effect on insulin levels, soy has also shown to significantly reduce androgens and oxidative stress in women with PCOS (22, 23, 24).

The research between soy intake and Hashimoto's, however, is inconsistent. Soy contains high amounts of phytoestrogens, a plant-derived compound known to have similar functions to human estrogen but with much weaker effects. Some test tube studies have demonstrated that phytoestrogens inhibit production of T3 and T4 thyroid hormones. Furthermore, one small human study found that phytoestrogen supplementation, at a level reflecting that found in a vegetarian diet, had a detrimental effect on thyroid status in patients with hypothyroidism (25). A different study of patients with hypothyroidism using a higher dose of phytoestrogen did not find any changes in thyroid status. Overall, a large review of all studies on the effects of dietary phytoestrogens on hormone levels in humans concluded that soy intake may negatively affect thyroid function in people with hypothyroidism (26).

Why We Recommend Eliminating Soy in Month Two

Soy has various health benefits, especially for women with PCOS, which is why we don't recommend a blanket soy-free diet for all patients. However, there are a few reasons why we suggest a temporary soy elimination in month two. First of all, like gluten and dairy, some people may not tolerate soy products (at first or at all). This food sensitivity isn't necessarily related to the soy itself, but rather the health of your gut and overall immune system. Based on available research, we also know that soy intake may worsen thyroid function in people with hypothyroidism.

Growing conditions is another concern for consuming soy. More than 90 percent of the soy grown in the United States is genetically modified. These GMO crops are sprayed heavily with a weed-killing chemical called glyphosate that may affect reproduction, hormone balance, and the gut microbiome (27, 28, 29).

If you have lingering symptoms after month one, temporarily eliminating soy in month two may assist in healing the gut, reducing inflammation, and improving food tolerance. Many gluten-free products replace gluten with a soy derivative, so make sure to check ingredient lists for hidden sources of soy.

If you choose to keep soy in your diet, keep these factors in mind:

- Choose whole food sources, like soybeans or edamame. Avoid processed versions like soy protein isolate or soybean oil.
- Choose organically grown, non-GMO soy to reduce glyphosate residue.
- Avoid eating soy every day.

Since soy may have positive health benefits for women with PCOS, we'll explain how to trial reintroduction of this food to your diet in month three.

Corn

Similar to soy, corn is another fairly common food sensitivity that is also heavily sprayed with glyphosate. Whether it's from burgers and fries, salad dressings, sweetened beverages, or corn fed to the animals we eat, corn is pervasive in today's modern food supply. Corn is the last main food we recommend eliminating during month two.

Unfortunately, removing corn from your diet goes far beyond eliminating the obvious popcorn, corn tortillas, and corn-on-the-cob. Corn is ubiquitous in our food supply and used in many ways you would never suspect. Here are a few tips to help you remove corn from your diet this month:

- Avoid overly processed foods. If it comes in a package, double check the ingredient list to check for sources of corn.
- Be aware of potential corn by-products to avoid like dextrin, maltodextrin, maize, sorbitol, cornmeal or grits, hominy, and polenta.

- Consider replacing traditional grain-fed beef and pork for grass and pasture-raised alternatives.

If you choose to keep corn in your diet, choose organic and whole-food varieties.

Summary of Month Two

Month two is designed to build on top of the solid food and supplement foundation you created in month one. If you were not able to follow the month one program with more than 75 percent consistency, we encourage you to restart month one for the best results. If you were fairly consistent throughout month one, but your follow-up symptom survey indicated lingering issues, we recommend completing a temporary elimination diet during this second month.

In month two, you will continue to follow the recommendations of month one (Hormone Balancing Meal Plan plus recommended supplements) in addition to removing food sources of gluten, dairy, soy, and corn.

Month 3

The final month of our 3-month program is a gradual reintroduction of eliminated foods intended to assess your individualized reaction (or lack thereof). As a reminder, month two involved the temporary elimination of gluten, dairy, soy, and corn.

Before we get started, take a few minutes to complete your final symptom survey.

Compare this final symptom survey to your initial and secondary surveys. Compared to your second follow-up survey, did your overall score increase, decrease, or remain the same after removing gluten, dairy, soy, and corn?

Reintroducing Foods

The final month of our program is aimed to continue the food and supplement plan from month one while reintroducing food categories eliminated during month two. It is not necessary to reintroduce any of these foods if you wish to keep them out of your diet. However, when done correctly, food reintroduction is an effective way to determine which foods may or may not trigger a reaction.

Follow these tips to methodically reintroduce the four foods eliminated in month two (gluten, dairy, soy, and corn).

1. Only reintroduce one new food at a time.
2. Eat an unprocessed form of the food two to three times in the same day. For example, instead of eating a traditional hamburger from a fast food restaurant to reintroduce gluten, have a slice of whole-grain toast in the morning and include a ½ cup of whole-grain pasta for dinner.
3. Wait at least 48 hours to monitor for any reaction (you can use our Food Reintroduction - Symptoms Tracker below as a guide).
4. If there is no reaction to that food, you can keep that food in your food plan and continue with the next food for reintroduction.
5. If you are unsure whether or not you had a reaction, you can retest the same food in the same manner.

	Brain Fog	Mood	Digestion: Bloating, Diarrhea, Constipation	Headache	Fatigue	Joint Pain Muscle Aches	Skin Changes
Dairy							
Gluten							
Soy							
Corn							

Reintroduce 1 new food category every 3 days
Record symptoms for 48 hours after eating each food

Food reintroduction is a great way to tune into your body and truly assess how you are feeling! We trust that you know your body best. If you feel like a certain food just doesn't sit well with you, trust your intuition!

Moving Forward

We are so proud of you for making it this far! No matter what the previous three months may have looked like, you made a conscious decision to take charge of your health. Healing is not always glamorous and it definitely is not linear. You may experience multiple dips or valleys throughout your journey, but the most important factor is that you keep going. James Clear said it best in his bestselling book, Atomic Habits:

The same way that money multiplies through compound interest, the effects of your habits multiply as you repeat them. They seem to make little difference on any given day and yet the impact they deliver over the months and years can be enormous. It is only when looking back two, five, or perhaps ten years later that the value of good habits and the cost of bad ones becomes strikingly apparent.

Healing takes time and consistency, so aim for progress over perfection.

Key Takeaways

- The goal of our Root Protocol is to treat the five root causes, eliminate your related symptoms, and help you achieve hormonal harmony with sustainable changes.
- The first month of our 3-month plan includes a diet rehaul with our Hormone Balancing Meal Plan using PFC, the Root Plate, and targeted supplementation.
- Our Core Supplement Bundle includes inositol, NAC, omega-3, and magnesium. Optional supplements at this time include vitamin D, a B-complex vitamin, and zinc.
- Depending on your individual circumstances, the second month of our 3-month plan includes a temporary elimination of gluten, dairy, soy, and corn. You will also continue the Hormone Balancing Meal Plan and recommended supplements through month two.
- In the last month of our 3-month plan, you will gradually reintroduce these four foods to monitor for any reaction.

9

Gut Health Deep Dive

In chapter seven, we described one of the most influential root causes of PCOS and Hashimoto's: gut health. Jessica, our case study example, suffered from PCOS, IBS, and multiple related symptoms like acne, diarrhea, and anxiety. After conducting a functional stool test, we identified dysbiosis in her gut. By using a targeted gut health protocol, we are able to help patients, like Jessica, reverse their dysbiosis, reduce or eliminate symptoms, and possibly prevent development of auto-immune conditions, like Hashimoto's.

If you completed the food and supplement plan outlined in chapter eight but still have lingering and frustrating symptoms, these next two chapters are essential. Healing the gut is an extensive subject with an incredibly powerful effect on PCOS and Hashimoto's. Therefore, we dedicated an additional chapter for a deep dive into the functional gut health protocol we use in our practice.

The 5R Protocol

The 5R protocol is the functional medicine protocol we use to treat complex gut disorders from the root cause. This protocol involves five steps. While some of these steps you can do on your own, we highly recommend working with a skilled functional medicine provider to prevent you from wasting time or money on unnecessary or ineffective interventions.

Remove

The first step of the 5R protocol aims to remove any factors causing harm, inflammation, or imbalance within the gut. For example, in this step we may recommend gentle antimicrobial herbs to reduce bacterial overgrowth and remove pathogens (like parasites or Candida). We also want to remove any other sources of inflammation, like food sensitivities, so we may recommend temporarily eliminating gluten, dairy, soy, and corn from your diet. Other inflammatory foods we recommend eliminating during this time include foods that will disrupt gut health: added sugar, fast food, refined grains, and alcohol.

Let's review a few specific gut conditions which may require more targeted removal with the help of a functional medicine provider.

Food Sensitivities

Food sensitivities occur when your immune system reacts to a particular food. However, unlike food allergies, food sensitivity reactions are often delayed and dose-dependent. This means that a food you ate yesterday could cause unwanted symptoms today or even tomorrow.

Common symptoms of food sensitivities include:

- Abdominal pain or bloating
- Constipation or diarrhea
- Acid reflux
- Migraines
- Acne or eczema
- Chronic fatigue
- Depression
- Brain fog
- Flare of autoimmune symptoms

• Joint pain

Each person has an individualized response to food sensitivity reactions, so the list of potential symptoms is often quite long. In the first step of the 5R protocol, you will remove potential food sensitivities to begin healing the gut. You can do this in one of two ways. First, you can undergo a temporary elimination diet removing the most common food sensitivities: gluten, dairy, corn, and soy. We discussed these foods in chapter eight, so if you removed these foods during month two of the program, you are already ahead of the game! This is the most affordable way to address food sensitivities. In general, we recommend removing food sensitivities throughout the entirety of the 5R protocol (three months or longer). These are the foods you have identified as sensitivities after removing the food group for one month and then doing a trial re-introduction as described in the last chapter.

The second way you can remove food sensitivities is by identifying your personal food triggers through an individualized food sensitivity test. The Mediator Release Test (MRT) is the food sensitivity test we use at Root Functional Medicine because it captures all types of food sensitivity reactions. You can read more about MRT on our website at https://rootfunctionalmedicine.com/how-is-mrt-different-from-other-food-sensitivity-tests/.

We particularly recommend MRT and the food plan that follows it for Hashimoto's as we find a lot of success using this testing and food plan for calming inflammation associated with autoimmune disease.

Food sensitivities are not a root cause, but rather a symptom of an unresolved issue in your gut. Most often, food sensitivities are caused by dysbiosis, a leaky gut, and underlying inflammation (Figure 9.1). While removing food sensitivities is an important first step in healing the gut, we must also address the underlying causes of these food reactions.

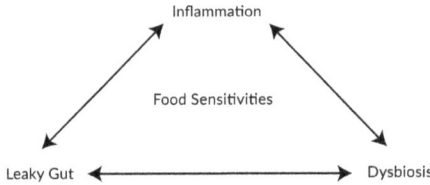

Figure 9.1

Dysbiosis

We talked about dysbiosis a lot in this book because it is a key player in the root cause of PCOS and Hashimoto's. As you know by now, dysbiosis is the overarching name for a general imbalance of gut bacteria. You may have too much "bad" bacteria, too little "good" bacteria, or not enough diversity of bacteria in your gut. Dysbiosis can be the genesis of the insulin resistance, high androgens, and inflammation seen in PCOS. What's more, dysbiosis may reduce your body's ability to convert T4 into the active T3 thyroid hormone thereby worsening hypothyroidism. In our practice, we use a functional stool test to diagnose dysbiosis in our patients. For this test, our patients collect an at-home stool sample and ship it to the laboratory with the provided mailing kit. This stool test looks for harmful bacteria, diversity of bacteria, parasites, inflammation, and more. With this information, we develop a targeted protocol to remove harmful bacteria or parasites.

Small Intestinal Bacterial Overgrowth (SIBO)

SIBO is the name of a specific kind of dysbiosis that occurs when too many bacteria end up in the small intestine. Normally, your small intestine is home to a relatively small number of bacteria. Most of your gut bacteria are supposed to live in your large intestine. Hypochlorhydria, or low stomach acid, is one of the main causes of SIBO. Without enough acid in your stomach, microbes can survive digestion, camp out in the small intestine and feast on your partially digested food.

SIBO can also be triggered from an episode of food poisoning or the stomach flu.The bacteria or virus from the illness releases a toxin into the GI tract that can damage the cells that control your "cleansing waves." These cleansing waves are muscular contractions responsible for sweeping away debris from the small intestine. When the cleansing waves are disrupted, you can develop SIBO. Common symptoms of SIBO include acne, eczema, constipation/diarrhea, bloating, anxiety, brain fog, allergies, and more. Gut symptoms of SIBO are classically bloating after eating, especially after eating foods like cruciferous veggies or beans that contain FODMAPs and stool changes including either diarrhea or constipation.

The most agreed upon test to diagnose SIBO is a breath test. For this test, you drink a specific syrup and then provide breath samples at various time intervals. The bacteria in your small intestine feed on the syrup and produce hydrogen and/or methane gas. If the levels of gas are higher than the provided threshold, this may indicate a SIBO diagnosis.

An experienced functional medicine doctor may also make the diagnosis based on clinical symptoms and patterns of dysbiosis and inflammation seen on microbiome stool testing.

Candida Overgrowth

Candida albicans is a yeast present in our digestive tracts as well as other areas in the body. For example, a vaginal yeast infection is an overgrowth of yeast in the vaginal tract, while thrush is an overgrowth of yeast in the mouth. When your gut is healthy, beneficial bacteria keep *Candida* at low amounts to prevent overgrowth. When you do not have enough beneficial bacteria for this task, *Candida* overgrowth may occur. *Candida* overgrowth is another specific type of dysbiosis and may present with similar symptoms like constipation, bloating, and acne or eczema. Vaginal yeast infections or thrush (a white "cottage cheese" coating on the tongue) may be due to underlying *candida* over-growth in the gut as well. We can detect *candida* overgrowth with a stool test and may recommend gentle antimicrobial herbs and/or biofilm enzymes to treat this condition.

While removing food sensitivities is something you may be able to accomplish well at home, finding other sources that need to be removed in the gut may require functional stool testing and a consultation with a functional medicine doctor. We find that nearly everyone with both PCOS and Hashimotos has dysbiosis, so we created a gut health bundle on our website that includes the three most common supplements we use in rebalancing gut dysbiosis. If SIBO is suspected, we also like our SIBO probiotic.

In conventional medicine, SIBO is often treated with two weeks of antibiotic. In our experience, most people end up having a relapse if this is the only treatment that they receive. It's important to complete the rest of the 5R protocol and treat underlying causes of SIBO to prevent recurrence.

Replace

The second step of the 5R protocol replaces everything your body needs for optimal digestion and gut health. In this step, we may address low stomach acid, replace digestive enzymes, and replete any nutrient deficiencies.

Digestive Enzymes

Your pancreas and small intestine both release digestive enzymes to break down food into absorbable components. However, dysbiosis or damage to the gut lining may prevent your body from producing enough digestive enzymes to properly absorb your food. Symptoms of inadequate digestive enzymes may include: bloating or cramping after meals, undigested food in your stool, and gas. Supplementing with digestive enzymes throughout your 5R protocol promotes optimal digestion and may help reduce your GI symptoms. The digestive enzymes we offer at Root provide bile extract (helpful for digesting fat), various digestive enzymes for protein and carbohydrates, and betaine hydrochloric acid to replace stomach acid.

Low Stomach Acid

When the food you eat enters into your stomach, the cells lining your stomach release hydrochloric acid (HCl). Stomach acid helps your body breakdown the protein, fat, and carbohydrates from your meal. It also kills off any harmful bacteria or viruses to protect your body from infection or bacterial overgrowth. Unfortunately, aging, stress, vitamin deficiencies, and certain medications may lead to low levels of stomach acid. Common symptoms of low stomach acid can include bloating, burping, gas, and (surprisingly) heartburn. It is crucial to address low stomach acid, because this condition can be a root cause of dysbiosis, SIBO, and vitamin deficiencies required for hormone balance.

The easiest way to determine if you have low stomach acid is to complete a HCl challenge. You can purchase HCl over-the-counter usually under the name "betaine HCl." This is best done under the direction of your physician. People with a history of ulcers or esophagitis should not take betaine.

Popular functional medicine protocols for doing a betaine challenge are:

Begin by taking one pill of betaine HCl with a protein-containing meal and observe how you feel:

- If you have discomfort or heartburn, you do NOT have low stomach acid.
- If you feel fine (or better than usual), take two capsules of HCl with each meal.

If you have no reaction with two pills per meal after two days, increase the number of HCl to three pills with each meal.

Continue increasing the number of HCl pills every two days to up to four pills with each meal (or as recommended by your healthcare provider).

You'll know if you have taken too much if you experience tingling, heartburn, or any other form of discomfort. When you reach this state of discomfort, cut back by one capsule per meal.

Your ideal dose is established once you have no symptoms of burning or discomfort. Keep in mind that you may require less HCl with smaller meals.

Typically, once gut health is restored, there is no longer a need for HCl supplements. Some digestive enzymes also contain a smaller dose of betaine than stand alone betaine capsules. Most individuals who take HCl while they are doing the 5R protocol then stop after completion of the gut healing protocol. Monitor your symptom improvement and attempt to cut back on HCl as you improve.

Nutrient Deficiencies

Individuals with impaired gut health often have multiple nutrient deficiencies due to prolonged malabsorption and/or eating the standard American diet (which lacks many important nutrients). The Supplement Bundle and optional supplements we recommended in chapter eight includes many of the most common nutrient deficiencies we see in women with PCOS and/or Hashimoto's: magnesium, omega-3, vitamin D, zinc, and a B-complex vitamin. Many of these nutrients are particularly helpful in the third step of the 5R protocol to repair the gut lining.

Repair

In the first two steps, we removed irritants to the gut microbiome and replaced factors essential for optimal digestion. The next step of the 5R protocol involves repairing damage to the intestinal wall. Your intestines contain a protective barrier, or lining, to prevent uncontrolled entry of undigested food, bacteria, and toxins from entering the body. It also prevents loss of water and electrolytes while allowing for proper absorption of nutrients. These intestinal cells are linked together by proteins called "tight junctions" which act as the gatekeepers to control what can or cannot enter the intestinal cells. When the integrity of the gut lining is compromised through dysbiosis, inflammation, or infection, larger food proteins or harmful bacteria may enter into the cell. This is known as a "leaky gut."

There are a few nutrients that are particularly effective in healing the gut lining. First of all, zinc carnosine is a nutrient with anti-inflammatory, antioxidant, and wound healing functions which has shown to repair the gut lining (1). Furthermore, glutamine is an amino acid, antioxidant, and the primary nutrient and energy source for the cells lining your intestinal tract. Glutamine supplementation may be beneficial for individuals with leaky gut by strengthening tight junctions (the gatekeepers of your intestinal cells) (2). Finally, we have talked a lot about vitamin D throughout this book. We know that individuals with PCOS and/or Hashimoto's are more likely to have a vitamin D deficiency. We also know that lower vitamin D levels are associated with insulin resistance, high androgen levels, and worsening hypothyroidism. Thankfully, vitamin D is a powerhouse nutrient with anti-inflammatory benefits for the gut lining while simultaneously regulating gut bacteria.

In our practice, we like to recommend our Gut Health Rebalance powder for the repair step of the 5R protocol. This powder contains zinc carnosine, glutamine, and other nourishing ingredients for the gut lining like deglycyrrhizinated licorice (DGL), slippery elm, and aloe vera extract.

Reinoculate

Once we remove bacterial overgrowth (first R), replace factors essential for proper digestion (second R), and repair the gut lining (third

R), we move onto the fourth step of the 5R protocol: reinoculate. In this step, we reintroduce beneficial bacteria to promote a healthy gut microbiome.

Fermented Foods

In this step, we recommend including fermented foods into your diet, like raw sauerkraut, kimchi, and kombucha. Here are a few ideas for how to include these probiotic-rich foods into your meals and snacks:

- Use kombucha in place of spritzer/sparkling water.
- Mix kombucha into a fun mocktail.
- Add sauerkraut to your morning eggs.
- Add kimchi to your tacos.
- Put kimchi or sauerkraut as a condiment on your burger.
- Stir kimchi into fried rice or stir fry recipes.

Heating or canning may kill the microbes present in fermented foods. For this reason, choose fermented foods available in glass jars in the refrigerated section of the grocery store.

Probiotic Supplements

At this time, we also introduce a targeted probiotic supplement. However, we do not recommend purchasing a random probiotic supplement from the drug store. Probiotics are much more nuanced than you may think, and taking the right one is essential to effectively reinoculating your microbiome (and not wasting your money). We have a few good choices for probiotics that we use at Root.

The first probiotic we often start with at Root is a soil-based probiotic called MegaSporeBiotic. As the name implies, soil-based probiotics are bacteria found in the soil which generally contain bacteria strains from the *Bacillus* family. These bugs are commonly referred to as spore-forming probiotics because they are encapsulated with a hard shell, or endospore, making them very stable and highly resistant to extreme conditions. Unlike traditional probiotics, soil-based probiotics are more likely to survive the harsh environment of your GI tract that would otherwise destroy bacteria.

Soil-based probiotics have many documented benefits. First of all, these probiotics regulate your gut microbiome and reduce dysbiosis. This is one big difference between soil-based and conventional probiotics. For instance, taking 20 billion colony forming units (CFU) of a traditional probiotic is simply a drop in the ocean compared to the rest of your estimated 100 trillion gut bacteria. What's more, typical probiotics do not usually eliminate or prevent the growth of harmful bacteria. Soil-based probiotics, however, can distinguish between "good" and "bad" bacteria and may reduce dysbiosis by crowding out and even secreting antimicrobials to kill off the bad bacteria. One study investigating the role of soil-based probiotics in patients with irritable bowel syndrome (which is essentially dysbiosis) reported that the patients in the probiotic group reported a significantly higher quality of life and lower symptom scores than those who received typical antibiotic treatment (3). Furthermore, one of the main *Bacillus* strains in MegaSpore-Biotic is known for its antioxidant producing abilities. As we know, antioxidants benefit many other root causes of PCOS and Hashimoto's like insulin resistance and mitochondrial dysfunction (oxidative stress). Soil-based probiotics may also repair the gut lining and reduce leaky gut. In fact, one study found that taking a soil-based probiotic for 30 days reduced leaky gut by up to 42 percent (4). In addition to reducing leaky gut, a different study found that taking a spore-forming probiotic for eight weeks reduced inflammatory markers by up to 55 percent (5).

When starting MegaSporeBiotic, start low and go slow to reduce side effects.

- Week 1: take 1 capsule every other day
- Week 2: increase to 1 capsule daily
- Week 3+: take 2 capsules daily

If you begin to experience side effects like abdominal cramping or loose stools, reduce your starting dose to a ½ capsule every other day.

The second probiotic we use often is our Root probiotic which includes several different strains that are helpful in maintaining a good balance of bacteria. This is more cost effective and we also find it helpful for diarrhea.

Note: if you introduce these probiotics as instructed, but your symptoms worsen, this can be an indication that you have underlying SIBO or other gut issue that has not yet been addressed. In this case, we recommend working with a functional medicine provider to seek further testing and treatment.

Prebiotics

Prebiotics are high-fiber foods that feed your beneficial gut bacteria so they can thrive in their newly established environment. During this step of the 5R process, we recommend focusing on increasing the amount of natural prebiotics in your diet like:

- Garlic
- Onions
- Asparagus
- Oats
- Apples
- Bananas
- Flaxseeds
- Berries
- Leafy greens
- Lentils
- Quinoa
- Beans

For recipes, please refer to the appendix at the end of this book. Remember to follow the PFC and Root Plate guidelines to ensure proper blood sugar balance when increasing these prebiotic foods.

It is also possible to take a prebiotic supplement, though use caution as many popular fiber supplements can lead to bloating. We use our Root Low Fodmap Prebiotic supplement to support microbial diversity.

Rebalance

The final step of the 5R gut health protocol is called rebalance. Gut health is not excluded from the negative effects of stress. In fact, some researchers argue that the negative effects of stress on the body are partially due to its harmful impact on gut bacteria. For example, stress hormones increase the levels of harmful bacteria in the gut which eventually crowd out the beneficial bacteria. Studies looking at the microbiome of college students found that as stress increased throughout the semester, certain health-promoting bacteria decreased (6). By causing a state of dysbiosis, stress can also increase leaky gut. A Leaky gut allows bacteria to seep into circulation and produces an inflammatory response. Bottom line: you cannot fully heal the gut until you recognize and address the stress in your life. Ignoring stressors, like poor sleep, too much (or not enough) exercise, hectic schedules, and not enough self-care will wreak havoc on your gut, PCOS, and Hashimoto's. You can't eliminate stress from your life, but you can learn how to manage it! Stress is such an important part of healing from PCOS and Hashimoto's that we dedicated the next chapter to identifying, coping, and treating the negative effects of stress in your life.

Key Takeaways

- The 5R protocol is the functional medicine approach we use in our clinical practice to address underlying gut issues that cause PCOS and Hashimoto's.
- The first step of the 5R protocol removes any factors causing harm, inflammation, or imbalance within the gut. In this step, we eliminate food sensitivities, added sugar, and treat any forms of dysbiosis.
- The second 5R replaces everything your body needs for optimal digestion and gut health. In this step, we may replace low stomach acid with HCl, supplement with digestive enzymes, and replete any nutrient deficiencies.
- The third step of the 5R protocol repairs damage to the intestinal wall to reverse leaky gut. We usually recommend our Gut Health Rebalance power which contains ingredients known to heal the gut lining like zinc carnosine and glutamine.
- The fourth 5R is to reinoculate the gut with beneficial bacteria. In this step, we recommend introducing fermented foods, a targeted probiotic, and prebiotic-rich foods.
- The last step of the 5R protocol is designed to rebalance your life by reducing and managing physical or psychological stressors.

10

Adrenal Health Deep Dive

Stress is a normal reaction to everyday pressures. In some cases, stress can be a brief and positive force to influence motivation and performance. Yet, over time, chronic exposure to stress without relief negatively impacts your health and well-being. The American Psychological Association calls stress a "national mental health crisis." Although, stress impacts more than your mind. Your digestive tract, reproductive system, thyroid health, immune system, and more are all negatively affected by chronic stress. Women with PCOS and Hashimoto's are particularly vulnerable to the harmful consequences of stress. After adjusting for BMI, infertility, and socio-demographic factors, one study reported higher levels of perceived stress in women with PCOS than women without this condition (1). Another study showed that over 50 percent of participants with PCOS reported high or extremely high levels of stress (2). These individuals are also three times more likely to suffer from depression and five times more likely to report anxiety symptoms (3).

Stress creates a vicious cycle in PCOS and Hashimoto's as people with these conditions often experience stress as a result of their symptoms; yet, stress can make the root causes of PCOS and Hashimoto's worse. In chapter five, we spoke about how your body uses the hypothalamus-pituitary-adrenal (HPA) axis to control your response to stress. Let's review the basics of this system.

The primary function of your HPA axis is to regulate your response to stress by controlling a stress hormone called cortisol. While cortisol is normally produced in varying levels throughout the day, the HPA axis regulates your "fight-or-flight" response. After a stressful event, the hypothalamus should sense high levels of cortisol in the blood and tell your pituitary and adrenal glands to slow cortisol production. This exists so that your body does not produce excess cortisol after the stressful event is over. HPA axis dysfunction occurs when you live in a state of chronic stress and the communication from your brain to your adrenal glands is disrupted. Over time, this deranged feedback leads to either high or low cortisol levels. Imbalanced cortisol levels can have devastating side effects like insomnia, depression, low libido, irritability, weight gain (especially in the midsection), and fatigue.

When the adrenal glands release cortisol, they also inadvertently produce DHEA-S, a steroid hormone made by the adrenal glands. While DHEA-S does not do much on its own, it is converted into other powerful hormones like testosterone. High levels of DHEA-S are seen in about 25 percent of PCOS patients (4). Stress is a major contributor to DHEA production, and chronic stress can cause high levels of this hormone. DHEA-S is often the only androgen found to be elevated on bloodwork in women with PCOS with an adrenal gland root cause. Unfortunately, women with adrenal PCOS often go years without a proper PCOS diagnosis because they may not have typical insulin resistance or high testosterone levels.

Stress and high cortisol levels also aggravate Hashimoto's by decreasing active T3 thyroid hormone and increasing reverse T3. Lower T3 levels with a high reverse T3 often results in worsening symptoms of hypothyroidism.

Simply put, you cannot afford to ignore the adverse effects of poor sleep and chronic stress if you have PCOS and/or Hashimoto's. In this chapter, we will provide you with more in-depth and actionable information on supporting your HPA axis by lowering stress levels and treating insomnia.

Managing Stress

As you consider how to lower your stress levels, think about the root cause approach. What is the root cause of your chronic stress? For some, it may be relationships, finances, or an overextended schedule with too little time for self-care. Because stress is a natural part of life, we need to find a productive way to reduce the effects of everyday stress on our bodies.

In this section, we will review a few ways to effectively reduce your stress levels. We recommend choosing one or two stress management strategies you can implement into your daily routine.

Gratitude Journal

There is a growing body of evidence on the benefits of gratitude. Gratitude is the appreciation of what is meaningful to you. Essentially, it is a general state of thankfulness and appreciation.

A review of the research will tell you that gratitude can:

- Improve overall well being
- Enhance happiness and positive emotions
- Increase self-esteem
- Reduce work-related stress
- Improve your sleep quality
- Reduce depressive symptoms

While there is no right or wrong way to practice gratitude, some people find keeping a gratitude journal helpful. This activity can take five minutes or less each day! Plus, at the end of the year, you can look back and read all the positive things you wrote down each day. Try to be as specific as possible with your statements, including both big and small aspects of your day.

Worry Journal

Have you ever vented to your spouse, friend, or parent when you were stressed or anxious? For some people, venting is a cathartic release of emotion. Although it may seem counterintuitive, creating a worry journal is one way to identify faulty patterns of thinking and gain perspective on the things making you stressed. To get started, make a list of everything you are worried about in a few minutes. After the timer is up, go back and reflect on each worry. What is the root cause of each worry? Are you worried about the issue you wrote down or something deeper? Is worrying about this thing productive or unproductive? Keeping a worry journal helps you examine how your thoughts and perceptions of a situation—not the situation itself—affect the way you feel.

Meditation

Meditation is a state of heightened awareness which connects the body and mind. The benefits of regular meditation include lowering stress and cortisol levels, improving anxiety and depression, and enhancing overall quality of life (5, 6). There are different types of meditation, but the most common form is referred to as mindfulness meditation. Jon Kabat-Zinn, the founder of the popular mindfulness-based stress reduction technique, defines mindfulness meditation as "the awareness that arises from paying attention, on purpose, in the present moment and non-judgmentally."

We believe that everyone can benefit from even small amounts of meditation, so we recommend implementing at least five minutes of meditation every day. Fortunately, there are many resources which provide guided mindfulness meditations like Headspace, Calm, and Ten Percent Happier. There are also numerous meditation videos available for free on YouTube.

Therapy

Stress, trauma, depression, and anxiety can all affect both your mental and physical health. Thankfully, attending therapy is less stigmatized nowadays, and many individuals with PCOS and Hashimoto's find various therapy interventions extremely helpful. In fact, one study found women with PCOS undergoing therapy combined with diet and lifestyle modifications lost more weight than women who only underwent diet and lifestyle changes (7). Essentially, if we want to treat the whole body, we can't ignore what is happening in your mind. Many insurance companies now cover therapy sessions with an in-network provider. If you feel like therapy may help you cope with your stress, mood disorder, and/or underlying trauma, consider checking with your insurance for coverage or exploring online therapy programs like Betterhelp and Talkspace.

Box Breathing

Box breathing is a simple, yet profound, stress reducing technique that relaxes the body, improves oxygenation, and grounds you in mindfulness.

1. Close your eyes.
2. Breathe in deeply through your nose while slowly counting to four in your head.
3. Gently hold your breath while counting to four.
4. Begin to slowly exhale for four seconds.

Repeat these steps as needed. Some people find box breathing particularly helpful before an event perceived as stressful (like an interview) or before bed to treat insomnia.

Time Outdoors

Spending time in nature reduces cortisol levels and improves your overall sense of well being. Tackle two birds with one stone by incorporating a short nature walk into your daily routine. Practice mindful awareness of your surroundings by noticing the different sights, sounds, smells, and feel of everything around you. Gardening is also scientifically proven to reduce depression and anxiety as well as improve life satisfaction and quality of life.

Movement

Moving your body throughout the day provides benefits not only for physical health but also for lowering stress levels and improving overall mental health. Make it a daily goal to move your body for at least 30 minutes each day. This can be all at once or broken up into smaller movement breaks. Set an alarm to remind you to move during your day. Get outside for some fresh air, stretch, and step away from your computer at lunch! If you do not have a regular exercise routine established, start with this daily movement goal. From there, we encourage you to consider adding a more intentional exercise plan to your week. For example, strength training 2-3 times a week helps to build muscle and improves insulin resistance. High-intestinal interval training (HIIT) has also shown to improve insulin resistance; however, avoid doing HIIT every day as this will raise cortisol levels.

You may also consider syncing your exercise regimen with your menstrual cycle. For example, during your menses week, aim for more restorative movement, like yoga or walking. During your follicular phase, rising estrogen gives you more energy, which allows for more HIIT exercises. After ovulation, your luteal phase is a great time to incorporate more strength training. Finally, in the week before your period, consider adding more aerobic exercises like jogging, cycling, or the elliptical to promote the release of serotonin and other relaxing chemicals.

Schedule in Self-Care

If you want to treat the root cause of your PCOS and Hashimoto's, you have to make self-care and stress management a priority in your life. This may look like blocking out your calendar every day for 10 minutes while you practice meditation. Or, it may require you to leave your house 10 minutes earlier in order to practice box breathing in the car before heading into work or picking up your child from school. Take some time right now to brainstorm how you can arrange your schedule to make time for at least one of these stress-reducing techniques.

Sleep Quantity and Quality

Sleep is a complex and active restoration process for the body. Approximately one-third of your lifetime is spent asleep! Unfortunately, self-reported sleep times have decreased significantly in the past 50 years and up to 30 percent of Americans report sleeping less than six hours per night. Sleep dysfunction can have devastating effects on PCOS and Hashimoto's and worsens many of the root causes of these conditions, like insulin resistance, mitochondrial health, and HPA dysfunction. Sleeping less than six hours a night may also increase levels of CRP, a marker for inflammation. Plus, sleep deprivation causes an imbalance in your appetite hormones leaving you constantly hungry and never satisfied the next day. In fact, sleep deprivation may cause an estimated 40 percent increase in sugar cravings, and studies show people will eat around 300 more calories when sleep deprived versus when they are well rested.

Implementing positive sleep habits is crucial to setting a healthy foundation for sleep quality, quantity, and reducing insomnia. Here are a few general sleep hygiene tips we recommend implementing as soon as possible. We will dive deeper into a few of these tips throughout this chapter as well.

- **Skip the nightcap.** Despite what you may have heard, a drink before bed does not improve your sleep quality. While it may make you feel sleepy, alcohol actually fragments your sleep and causes frequent wakings throughout the night (even if you don't remember). Alcohol also strongly reduces restorative REM sleep.

- **Eliminate afternoon caffeine.** The half-life of caffeine is 6 to 8 hours (more or less depending on your genetics). So, if you drink coffee at 1pm, half of that caffeine may still be present in your bloodstream by 9 pm making it harder for you to relax before bed.
- **Avoid electronics before bed.** We will discuss this more in the melatonin section.
- **Establish a regular bedtime and routine.** The human body craves consistency and routine. We respect this innate desire with babies by creating a relaxing bedtime routine at a consistent time each night. However, as adults, we often forget the importance of these actions for a good night's sleep.
- **Keep your bedroom dark and cool.** The best temperature to induce sleep is 65-68 degrees fahrenheit. Block out any light to avoid sleep disruption.
- **Spend 30 minutes in natural sunlight.** Morning exposure is particularly beneficial in balancing your circadian rhythm.

In addition to the insomnia treatments we will discuss in the next sections, research also supports mind-body interventions, like yoga or tai chi, in reducing insomnia severity and improving sleep quality. Meditation and mindfulness exercises may also help reduce insomnia.

Supplements may also improve insomnia and sleep quality. Our favorite supplement for sleep is our Magnesium glycinate that is included in our PCOS bundle. Taking 200-300mg about 30 minutes before bedtime can be very helpful for sleep.

Sleep Apnea

Sleep apnea is a serious sleep disorder in which breathing stops repeatedly, sometimes hundreds of times, throughout the night. Untreated sleep apnea causes loud snoring and daytime fatigue even if you think you're getting a full night's sleep. This condition has devastating consequences if left untreated. For example, sleep apnea is associated with depression, high blood pressure, heart failure, high cholesterol and blood sugar levels, and weight gain or difficulty losing weight. Sleep apnea is diagnosed by detecting how many times you stop breathing at night during a sleep study. Individuals with PCOS have a greater incidence of sleep apnea compared to women without PCOS. While obesity is a strong risk factor for sleep apnea, this condition occurs in women with PCOS who have a BMI in the normal range as well (8).

Common symptoms of sleep apnea may include:

- Loud snoring
- Sore or dry throat upon waking
- Restless sleep
- Sleepiness during the day
- Morning headaches

If you have PCOS and suffer from any of these symptoms, we encourage you to speak with your doctor to see if they recommend a referral for a sleep study.

Hormones Affecting Sleep

Some hormone imbalances worsen sleep if left untreated. In this section, we will discuss two specific hormones that affect sleep: melatonin and progesterone.

Melatonin

Melatonin is a hormone released by your brain to regulate your circadian rhythm and synchronize your sleep-wake cycle with night and day. In humans, melatonin starts to release into the bloodstream about two hours before your regular bedtime and peaks around 3 am. Melatonin is not only a sleep regulator. It also acts as an antioxidant and is involved in egg quality and fertility. Egg quality is important even if you are not trying to get pregnant because the quality of your egg determines the health of your overall menstrual cycle. Here are a few ways to promote healthy melatonin levels:

Establish a regular bedtime and stick to it

Melatonin likes consistency, and your brain will trigger its release around two hours before it suspects bedtime. Training your brain to go to bed at the same time every night will help time this release.

Avoid electronics one to two hours before bed

We know this is so hard! However, blue light on electronic devices is known to significantly suppress melatonin release. Try charging your phone out of arm's reach at night and reaching for a printed book instead of your phone or tablet. Some smartphones have optional screen time restrictions you can set into place as well. For example, you can set a screen time limit to restrict use of social media apps after 8 pm. If restricting blue light exposure for two hours before bedtime seems unrealistic at this time, start small. Eliminating electronics even thirty minutes before bed can support a healthier melatonin release.

Get outside during the day

The rhythmic release of melatonin is regulated by a part of your brain called the suprachiasmatic nucleus (SCN). The SCN relies on cues from your environment to make adjustments to your circadian clock. For example, when you fly across multiple time zones, your circadian rhythm becomes out of sync with the time of your destination. The SCN relies on cues it receives through the retina in your eyes for adjustment. Exposing yourself to natural sunlight in the morning helps your SCN sync your circadian rhythm and melatonin for good quality sleep. During winter months, using a light box for 30-60 minutes in the morning can help to reset melatonin cycles as well.

Balance Estrogen Levels

Hormones work together to promote optimal balance in the body. When one hormone is disrupted, it often causes disruption to other downstream hormones as well. For example, estrogen is required to make serotonin (your "happy hormone"). Serotonin is required to make melatonin. If you do not have enough estrogen, you cannot make enough serotonin or melatonin. This estrogen deficiency is often the cause of insomnia in menopausal women. However, premenopausal women in their reproductive years can still suffer from low estrogen levels. Some causes of low estrogen include excessive exercise, extreme dieting, and autoimmune conditions.

Melatonin Supplements

Melatonin is a common supplement used to reduce symptoms of insomnia. As an antioxidant, a few studies found melatonin to have a beneficial effect on regulating ovulation in women with PCOS as well. However, melatonin (and supplements in general) should never be a substitute for healthy habits, good sleep hygiene, and addressing the root cause.

Progesterone

Does your insomnia worsen a few days before your period? It could be due to a progesterone deficiency. Progesterone is a reproductive hormone released after ovulation. Progesterone prepares the body for a potential pregnancy in the event that the released egg is fertilized. If the egg is not fertilized, progesterone production falls and a new menstrual cycle begins. Progesterone is known as your calming hormone and has many benefits like lowering anxiety and promoting healthy sleep. There are a few causes of progesterone deficiency.

Anovulation

Anovulation (or a lack of ovulation) is a primary cause of progesterone deficiency. Anovulation is fairly common in PCOS and Hashimoto's and is usually the result of insulin resistance and/or high androgen levels. Irregular or absent periods are often an indication that you are not regularly ovulating. You need to ovulate in order to produce progesterone, so any intervention that promotes regular menstrual cycles with ovulation will also help correct this type of progesterone deficiency. Our 3-month plan described in chapter eight is the best place to start to encourage more regular ovulation. As you may recall, this plan focuses on blood sugar balance, gut health, lowering androgens, and reducing oxidative stress with anti-inflammatory foods and targeted supplements. As your menstrual cycles normalize and you begin to ovulate regularly, you will likely notice an improvement in your sleep as well.

Luteal Phase Deficiency

Some women regularly ovulate but suffer from a progesterone deficiency known as a luteal phase defect (LPD). The luteal phase is the second half of your menstrual cycle from the day of ovulation until menstrual bleeding. A healthy luteal phase should last around 12 to 16 days. Although experts have varying opinions on what officially qualifies as LPD, we have noticed in our clinic that women with luteal phases of 11 days or less often suffer from symptoms of progesterone deficiency like infertility, recurrent pregnancy loss, spotting before your period, insomnia, and more. HPA axis and mitochondrial dysfunction are two probable causes of LPD. For more targeted information on these two root causes, refer to chapters five and seven. While working towards addressing the root cause of this type of progesterone deficiency, we may also recommend a progesterone supplement taken during your luteal phase.

Hypothyroidism

Underlying conditions, like hypothyroidism, may also cause a progesterone deficiency. You need adequate amounts of thyroid hormone to produce progesterone. If you have insomnia and suspect low progesterone levels, we recommend asking your doctor to run a full thyroid panel to screen for Hashimoto's (or to obtain updated lab values if you already have this condition).

Progesterone Testing

If you suspect a progesterone deficiency, you can request a progesterone test from your OB GYN. Many OB GYN clinics order a blood test for progesterone on cycle day 21. This is great if you regularly ovulate on day 14 of your menstrual cycle. However, as you know, women with PCOS and Hashimoto's often experience irregular periods and may ovulate later than what is considered normal. In this case, we recommend testing progesterone about seven days after you confirm ovulation. In our clinic, we also use dried urine tests to evaluate progesterone status. You can confirm ovulation with ovulation predictor kits, which detects the surge of luteinizing hormone (LH) prior to ovulation. Alternatively, you can also track your menstrual cycle and learn how to confirm ovulation using basal body temperature and changes in cervical mucus. Taking Charge of Your Fertility is a great book if you would like to learn more about natural cycle tracking.

Note: Most forms of the birth control pill and other hormonal contraceptives prevent ovulation, so testing for progesterone would not be useful in this scenario.

Supplements to Support HPA Dysfunction

We use and recommend targeted supplements with the patients in our practice. At risk of sounding like a broken record, we must remind you that supplements are not a quick fix or replacement for stress management strategies and good quality sleep. Rather, we use supplements to fill in the gaps of your diet and lifestyle and support your journey to healing.

Adaptogens

Adaptogens are plants that help your body cope with the effects of stress and promote hormonal balance. Adaptogens function mainly by affecting the HPA axis in response to external stress (whether mental, physical, or biological). These substances have been used in Ayurvedic medicine for thousands of years.

Ashwagandha is one of the main adaptogens we use in our practice. This plant has powerful and proven anti-inflammatory benefits that may lower cortisol levels, reduce anxiety, and help treat insomnia (9, 10). It is also helpful for women with adrenal PCOS as it may lower DHEA-S levels as well. Individuals with Hashimoto's can also benefit from ashwagandha as this adaptogen may improve TSH, T3, and T4 levels (11). Most studies show positive benefits of ashwagandha when supplementing with about 300 mg two times per day.

Maca, or Peruvian ginseng, is a plant from the Brassica family (similar to broccoli, cauliflower, and other cruciferous vegetables) that may also have adaptogenic properties. Some small studies show maca has promising benefits for fertility, mood, and libido (12). The HPA supplement we often recommend to our patients provides about 150 mg of maca per day.

L-Theanine & GABA

Theanine is an amino acid that increases the levels of "happy" and "calming" neurotransmitters in the brain, like GABA, serotonin, and dopamine. As a neurotransmitter, GABA has stress-reducing and sleep enhancing effects. Taking a combination of L-theanine and GABA may help individuals fall asleep quicker and prolong sleep duration (13).

Magnesium

Magnesium is an essential mineral and electrolyte we must obtain from our diet; however, an estimated 68 percent of Americans consume less than the recommended levels per day. Magnesium has over 300 functions in the body and plays a crucial role in hormonal balance and supporting your HPA axis. We recommend magnesium as part of our Core Supplement Bundle (see chapter eight) because it has such a positive impact on our patients with PCOS and Hashimoto's.

Magnesium regulates the HPA axis and supplementation may reduce exaggerated cortisol responses. This potential effect may explain why magnesium supplementation is an effective adjunctive therapy for treating major depression and reducing anxiety symptoms (14). Magnesium supplementation may reduce anxiety-related PMS symptoms too.

If you did not incorporate a magnesium supplement during your 3-month plan, we encourage you to do so now. Magnesium supplements are available in a variety of forms, including magnesium oxide, citrate, or bisglycinate. Magnesium bisglycinate is the most universal form that is well absorbed and tolerated with minimal GI side effects. Plus, this form of magnesium is combined with an amino acid called glycine which works with brain chemicals, like GABA, to promote feelings of calm. Glycine may also improve sleep quality and promote a healthy circadian rhythm. If you suffer from chronic stress, insomnia, anxiety, or other mood disorders, we recommend taking 200 mg of magnesium bisglycinate every day.

Key Takeaways

- Women with PCOS and Hashimoto's are more likely to suffer from chronic stress, mood disorders, and sleep disturbances.

- Adopting at least one regular stress-reducing strategy into your daily routine can lower cortisol levels, boost your mood, and increase your overall quality of life.
- Implementing positive sleep habits is crucial to setting a healthy foundation for sleep quality, quantity, and reducing insomnia.
- If you suffer from insomnia, adjust your habits to support healthy melatonin release, seek further testing if you suspect low progesterone levels, and talk to your doctor about sleep apnea (if applicable).
- Supplements to support a healthy HPA axis by reducing stress and improving sleep quality and duration include adaptogens, L-theanine and GABA, and magnesium.

11

Conclusion

PCOS and Hypothyroidism are two seemingly complex conditions involving multiple hormones, but which are actually joined and treatable at common root causes.

In this book we reviewed important steps to treat both conditions at root causes by addressing:

- Gut health
- Adrenal health and stress
- Blood sugar balance
- Replacing key nutrients
- Optimizing your environment

We have seen these methods work to restore regular periods even after women have gone years without a period. They have worked to achieve natural pregnancy even after failed IVF, or being told IVF would be needed. They have worked to improve brain fog, energy, mood, and improve thyroid function even after medication did not optimize.

You can do this too. Let this book be your guide for sustainable nutrition, appropriate supplementation, and knowing when it's time to dig further for root causes through testing and consultation with a functional medicine doctor and dietitian.

Helpful Resources:

The following appendices offer more resources to get you started including easy recipes following our Root Plate method and a supplement schedule that you can personalize based on your needs and preferences. Supplements can be found on the rootfunctionalmedicine.com Shop page or through your health care practitioner.

Resources for finding a functional medicine clinician near you include "find a practitioner" search on IFM.org. This is the Institute of Functional Medicine's database.

When ordering functional medicine testing, it is important to work with a professional who knows how to interpret these tests. However, there are several options depending on the state where you live to be able to order these tests directly on your own if your doctor does not have access to functional testing. We advise checking with your doctor first to make sure you will be able to take the results to them for interpretation. These direct ordering options include directlabs.com, ultalabs.com and Quest Diagnostics.

As you begin your steps to reversing your PCOS and thyroid symptoms at the root cause, remember that healing is a journey with ups and downs. Celebrate the small wins, be kind to yourself at setbacks and keep going one step at a time.

RESOURCES

Breakfast

All the breakfast recipes will also work for month 2 if you proceed with the temporary elimination of dairy, corn, gluten, and soy.

Smoothie Formula: 1 - 1.5 cups fruit + 1-2 healthy fat sources + 1-2 protein sources + 2 handfuls of greens + liquid
Healthy Fat: seeds, nuts, nut butter, coconut, coconut oil, avocado
Protein: collagen, hemp seed protein powder, pumpkin seed protein powder, pea protein
Optional add-ins: Cocoa powder, cinnamon, ginger, turmeric, any supplement powders (such as inositol or gut health powders)

Smoothies all make 1 serving.

Chocolate Cherry Smoothie
1 cup frozen cherries
1/2 banana
1/4 cup frozen riced cauliflower
1-2 large handfuls of leafy greens (spinach, baby kale,or chard)
1 tbsp cocoa powder
1 tbsp almond butter or peanut butter
1-2 scoops collagen or other single-ingredient protein powder
8-12 oz liquid (water or plant-based milk)

Basic Green Smoothie

1 cup tropical fruit (mango or pineapple)
1-2 large handfuls of leafy greens (spinach, baby kale, or chard)
2 tbsp of seeds (chia, ground flax, or hemp)
1-2 tsp of coconut oil
1-2 scoops collagen or other single-ingredient protein powder
8-12 oz liquid (water or plant-based milk)

Blueberry Banana Smoothie
½ frozen banana* (more on the green side)
1 cup frozen blueberries (or any type of berry)
1-2 large handfuls of leafy greens (spinach, baby kale, or chard)
1-2 tbsp nut butter of choice (peanut, almond, cashew, etc.)
2 tbsp of seeds (chia, ground flax, or hemp)
1-2 scoops of single-ingredient protein powder
8-12 oz liquid (water or plant-based milk)

How to make them: Combine all ingredients in a blender and blend for 30-60 seconds until it reaches desired consistency. You might need to add more liquid depending how frozen your ingredients are.

Egg Bake with Sausage & Greens
This is a great meal prep recipe to make ahead.
Makes 6-8 servings

Ingredients:

- 12 eggs
- 1 lb ground turkey, chicken, or pork sausage
- 1/2 onion, diced
- 1 bell pepper, diced
- 4-6 large handfuls of greens (spinach, kale, or chard)*

- Avocado oil or olive oil cooking spray
- Salt, to taste
- Pepper, to taste
- Desired spices (garlic powder, oregano, parsley, etc.)
- Optional: freshly grated cheese **(omit if eliminating dairy)**

How to make it: Brown the sausage with the onion and pepper. When it is almost done cooking, throw the greens on top to steam. Cover the pan with a lid. Spray a 9x13" pan with avocado oil or olive oil cooking spray. Spread the cooked sausage and greens over the bottom of the pan. In a bowl, whisk the eggs. Add salt, pepper, and other seasonings as desired. Pour the eggs over the sausage and greens. Bake at 350F for 40-60 minutes or until the eggs are fully cooked. *You can also use frozen chopped greens and skip steaming. Mix the frozen chopped greens into the bowl with eggs and pour over sausage.

Serve with: 1 serving fresh fruit. This gives you your "starch" component of the Root Plate (not technically a starch but this is where fruit would go on the Root plate).

Overnight Oats
Makes 1 serving

Ingredients:
- ¼ cup old fashioned rolled oats (GF if needed)
- 1 tbsp chia seeds
- 1 tbsp ground flaxseeds (flaxseed meal)
- 1 tbsp hemp seeds
- 1 scoop collagen or plant-based protein powder*
- 1 tsp pure maple syrup or honey (optional)
- ¼-⅓ cup liquid (water or plant-based milk)

Optional flavor add-ons: cocoa powder, cinnamon, ginger, pumpkin spice

Toppings:
• 2 tbsp nuts or other seeds (walnuts, pecans, slivered almonds, pumpkin seeds) or nut butter
• 1⁄2 cup berries**

How to make it: Combine all ingredients (except toppings) in a wide-mouth mason jar or bowl with a lid and stir well to combine. Cover and place in the refrigerator overnight (or for at least 4 hours). When ready to eat, enjoy cold or heat in the microwave. Top with nuts and berries in the morning. You can make several jars at once and eat throughout the week!

*Adding protein to oats is essential for keeping blood sugar balanced. You could also have 1-2 hard boiled or fried eggs on the side for protein if you choose not to add protein powder to your oats.

**Pro-tip: You can also put frozen berries in the jar and let them unthaw with the oats overnight.

Chia Pudding
Makes 1 serving

Ingredients:
• 3⁄4 cup plant-based milk
• 1⁄4 cup chia seeds
• 1⁄2 tbsp pure maple syrup (optional)
• 1-2 scoops of collagen or plant-based protein powder*

Toppings:
• Add 1-2 tablespoons of pumpkin seeds (pepitas), walnuts, or slivered almonds for texture.
• Otional: Nut butter, fresh berries

How to make it: Combine all ingredients (except toppings) in a wide-mouth mason jar or bowl with a lid and stir well to combine. Cover and place in the refrigerator overnight (or for at least 4 hours). You may want to give the chia seed pudding a stir after about 30 minutes to make sure everything is well combined. The texture in the morning should be thick and creamy. Add toppings in the morning. You can make several jars at once and eat throughout the week!

Optional add-ins (before refrigerating): Pure cocoa powder, frozen fruit, cinnamon, vanilla extract.

*Protein is important for blood sugar regulation

Lunch & Dinner Recipes

Slight modifications to the recipes are noted if applicable to fit the elimination diet in month 2.

Chicken & Apple Salad
Ingredients:
• 2-3 cups mixed greens
• 3 oz cooked chicken, sliced
• Apple*, thinly sliced
• 2 tbsp chopped walnuts
• 2 tbsp sunflower seeds
Optional: 1-2 tbsp feta cheese (cow's or goat's milk) (**Omit if eliminating dairy**)

Ingredients for Salad Dressing:
• 1-2 tbsp extra virgin olive oil

- 1 tbsp apple cider vinegar
- 1/2 tbsp pure maple syrup or honey
- 1 tsp Dijon mustard
Salt & pepper to taste (optional)

How to make it: Build salad with mixed greens, chicken, apples, walnuts, and sunflower seeds. For dressing, place all ingredients in a jar and shake to combine. Toss salad with dressing.

*You can use any type of apple. Keep the skin on for extra fiber. You also can use berries or whatever fruit you desire for this recipe.

Easy Salmon Cakes
Serving size: 2 salmon cakes.
Recipe makes around 3 servings.

Ingredients:
2-(6 oz) cans of boneless/skinless wild-caught salmon*
1/2 -2/3 cup almond flour or chickpea flour
2 eggs
Seasonings of choice: garlic powder, salt, pepper, oregano, or dill (add at least 1 teaspoon of 2-3 of these)
Avocado oil, olive oil, or ghee, for frying.

How to make it: Combine in the same bowl: 12 oz of salmon, 2 eggs, 1/2 - 2/3 cup of almond flour or chickpea flour as a binder, and seasonings of choice. Mix all ingredients together and form into 6 patties. Pan-fry the patties in a small amount of avocado oil (just enough to keep from sticking to the pan, not a "deep fry") for 3-4 minutes per side or until golden brown.

Serve with: Serve the salmon cakes with half of a plate of frozen or roasted vegetables and/or over rice or cauliflower rice.

Optional (but highly recommended!): Top with a homemade tartar sauce made using avocado oil based mayonnaise mixed with pickles + garlic + lemon juice.

*You can also use 12 oz of freshly cooked and shredded salmon

Egg Roll in a Bowl
Makes about 4 servings
Ingredients:
• 2 bell peppers, diced
• 1 white onion, diced
• 1-2 cups shredded carrots (okay to buy pre-shredded)
• 1-2 cups shredded cabbage (okay to buy pre-shredded)
• 1-2 tbsp avocado oil
• 1-2 tbsp sesame oil
• 4 tbsp coconut aminos
• 1 lb ground chicken, beef, pork, or turkey
• 2 cups cooked rice or quinoa
• 1/4 cup scallions
• 1/2 cup cilantro
• 2 tablespoons sesame seeds
• Sriracha or hot sauce, optional

How to make it: In a skillet, cook ground meat until thoroughly cooked. While the pork is cooking, dice the peppers and onion. Once the pork is cooked, place the pork in a bowl and heat more avocado oil in the skillet. Add peppers, onion, carrots, and cabbage. Sauté, s:rring occasionally. When the vegetables are beginning to soften, add the meat back in. Add sesame oil and coconut aminos and mix everything well.

Serve with: Rice, quinoa, or cauliflower rice. Top with scallions, cilantro, sesame seeds, and sriracha or hot sauce if you like more spice (optional).

Taco Salad Bowl
Makes 3-4 servings

Ingredients:
- 1-2 heads romaine lettuce, chopped
- 1 lb ground beef or turkey
- 1 small onion, diced
- 1 colored bell pepper, diced
- 2-4 garlic cloves, minced
- Taco seasoning*, 1 packet (you can also make your own)
- 1 can black beans, drained and rinsed
- Salsa
- Avocado**

How to make it: Brown ground beef in pan with onion, garlic, & bell pepper. Add taco seasoning. While beef is cooking, chop up the head of romaine. Assemble taco salad bowl with romaine lettuce on the bottom, 1/2 cup of black beans, a scoop of taco meat with onion and pepper. Top with salsa and avocado and use this in place of traditional salad dressing.
Serve with:
Toppings (optional)
- Cilantro
- Freshly shredded cheese **(omit if eliminating dairy)**
- Hot sauce
- Grain-free tortilla chips **(avoid corn in ingredients if eliminating)** (a small amount crunched on top)

• Pepitas

Quick guacamole recipe: Mash avocado and squeeze in lime juice + garlic + salt.**

*Depending on the brand of taco seasoning you are using, it may contain soy, gluten, or corn. Be aware of this during month 2.

Easy Anti-inflammatory Slow Cooker Chicken Soup
Makes about 4 servings
Ingredients:

- 6 cups of chicken bone broth
- 1 medium onion, diced 3 large carrots, peeled & diced
- 3 celery ribs, diced
- 2 cups of diced potatoes (gold or red)
- 1 lb boneless, skinless chicken thighs
- 1 tablespoon of thyme
- 1 tablespoon of rosemary
- 1 tablespoon of parsley
- 1 tablespoon of oregano
- 1 tablespoon of grated ginger
- 2 teaspoons of ground or fresh turmeric root
- 4-6 cloves of minced garlic
- 1/2 tsp pepper
- • Salt to taste (likely 1-2 tsp, depending how much salt is in the broth you are using) •
- 4 cups of chopped Swiss chard or kale

How to make it: Place all ingredients except for the leafy greens and chicken into the crockpot. Stir well. Place the chicken thighs into the crockpot and make sure they are submerged in the broth. Cook on high for 3-4 hours or low for 6-8 hours. About 1 hour before the end of cooking, taste the broth and add additional seasoning to suit your taste (if necessary). If the chicken is done, shred at this time with 2 forks (either right in the crockpot, or remove it and shred it on a plate and then place it back in the crockpot). At the end of cooking, stir in the 4 cups of leafy greens and let wilt into the soup for around 10 minutes before serving.

Serve with: A small side salad topped with seeds and a vinaigrette!

Other options: Add Squeeze of fresh lemon juice at the end of cooking.

Salmon, Sweet Potato, & Brussels Sprouts Sheet Pan Dinner
Makes 2 servings
Ingredients:

- 2 salmon filets
- 1 medium sweet potato, diced
- 4 cups Brussels sprouts, halved
- Avocado oil
- Garlic powder
- Salt
- Pepper
- Sesame seeds
- Dill (fresh or dried)
- Juice of 1 lemon

How to make it: Season salmon with sesame seeds, dill, and squeeze of lemon juice. Place on one end of a medium baking sheet. Toss diced sweet potato in avocado oil and season with garlic, salt, and pepper. Place in the middle section of the baking sheet. Lastly, toss Brussels sprouts in avocado oil and season with garlic, salt, and pepper. Place on the remaining section of the baking sheet. Roast at 400F for about 15-20 minutes until the salmon is fully cooked and vegetables are tender.*

*Root vegetables often take the longest to cook. You could begin roasting these first, or remove protein and continue roasting the vegetables until tender. Dicing potatoes smaller than other vegetables can be helpful. You can also microwave potatoes and then chop and add to the sheet pan.

Snacks

Slight modifications to this list may be needed if you are following the elimination diet in month 2.

1 clementine + handful of walnuts

½ cup raspberries + 1-2 hard boiled eggs

Carrot/pepper strips + hummus or guacamole

1 oz 70% dark chocolate + 1 tablespoon of nut butter

Plain Full-Fat Greek Yogurt + ¼ cup strawberries + 1 tablespoon ground flax

Plantain chips + guacamole

Grass-fed beef jerky

2 cups organic popcorn popped in coconut oil + salt + pepitas mixed in

Sardines + almond flour or seed crackers

Rice cake + almond butter + blueberries, hemp seeds, & cinnamon

2 tablespoons sunflower seeds + 2 brazil nuts + 1 tablespoon dark chocolate chips

No-Recipe Meals

We realize it's not always feasible to follow a recipe for every meal based on time and place and what you have on hand. We want to empower you to be able to put together your own meals to help you be successful in the long term. Here is some inspiration.

Breakfast:

Fry 2-3 eggs in avocado oil or ghee, wilt 2 cups of spinach in with the eggs at the end of cooking and season with salt, pepper, and/or everything bagel seasoning. Serve with 1 cup of fresh berries.

Full-fat, plain Greek yogurt or Skyr **(omit if eliminating dairy)** (look for grass-fed, organic if possible) + 1-2 tablespoons of chia, flax, or hemp seeds + fresh berries + sprinkled with chopped walnuts. Sub full-fat coconut milk yogurt for dairy-free and consider adding protein powder to get breakfast to 20 grams of protein.

Breakfast hash with sauteed sweet potatoes, chicken sausage, onions, peppers, and seasonings of choice

Dinner leftovers! You do not need to eat "breakfast" foods for breakfast.

Lunch & dinner:

Tuna mixed with avocado oil mayo, dijon mustard, chopped onions, celery, radishes, cucumber + desired seasonings served over a bed of greens with almond flour crackers or fruit. You could also mix the tuna with hummus and top with avocado.

Pre-chopped vegetable salad kit (such as chopped Brussel's sprouts, kale, and cabbage) with pre-cooked chicken + homemade vinaigrette dressing.

Small baked potato with ghee or grass-fed butter **(omit if eliminating dairy)** served with half of a plate of frozen broccoli and 2-3 fried eggs on top. Season as desired.

Bell peppers stuffed with seasoned meat & veggies and roasted in the oven until tender.

Meal Prep Ideas

- Start with the meal that is hardest for you. For some people this is breakfast, since mornings can be so rushed, for others it is lunch, etc.
- Egg bake, overnight oats, chia pudding, and crockpot meals are all excellent options to prep ahead.
- Wash and cut up vegetables to use in stir fry, roast, etc throughout the week (or use frozen!)
- Cook a starch source ahead of time (bonus: cooking and cooling potatoes or rice increases the resistant starch the feeds good bacteria in the gut).
- Roast a sheet pan of veggies.

- Throw chicken into the crock pot with some broth and seasonings and shred once fully cooked to eat with various things during the week.

How to roast any veggie:

It's going to take some experimenting but almost all veggies taste great roasted! Chop veggies to equal size pieces. Toss in avocado oil and add desired spices (salt, pepper, garlic powder, oregano, etc.) and roast on 400 degrees F for 20-30 minutes until golden brown and tender. Start checking on them and give them a stir after about 15 minutes

Formula for homemade vinaigrette:

1-2 tbsp extra virgin olive oil
1 tbsp apple cider vinegar or lemon juice
½ tbsp honey or pure maple syrup (optional)
1 tsp Dijon mustard
Place all ingredients in a jar and shake to combine.

This is a sample schedule of supplements that can naturally support hormone balance and blood sugar balance and replete essential nutrients for egg quality and thyroid function.

Check with your doctor to see if these will work with any of your existing medications or if you are pregnant or nursing. The supplements themselves can be combined safely together.

Root PCOS Bundle Supplements:

Supplement	Uses and conditions	Dose
Inositol (2,000mg myo-inositol and 50mg D-chiro-inositol)	A sugar made in the body and found in food. Improves menstrual regularity, egg quality, and fertility in women with PCOS. It can also help reduce cholesterol levels and TSH and improve insulin sensitivity.	One with breakfast and one with dinner.

NAC (N-acetyl-cysteine)	An antioxidant that may lower inflammation. Comes from the amino acid cysteine. Helps with blood sugar balance, mood, and supports liver detoxification.	900mg with breakfast and 900mg with dinner.
Magnesium glycinate	A mineral. Supports relaxation, sleep, and stress as well as hormone and blood sugar balance.	200-300mg 30 minutes before bedtime
Omega 3 (Fish Oil)	Important fats obtained from the diet. The most bioavailable and usable Omega 3s are animal based. Supports the immune system, mood, hormones, and may lower inflammation.	800-1000mg once daily

Key Nutrients:

Other key nutrients include zinc and vitamin D. It is helpful to know your lab values of these, however these are the most common doses. Zinc is helpful to add for 3 months to improve acne.

Vitamin D	A fat soluble vitamin that supports the immune system, energy, and mood.	2,000 IUs once daily (more may be required if deficient)

Zinc	A nutrient found most commonly in meat and seafood. Many on vegetarian diets are deficient. Supports the immune system, ovulation, and skin health	20-30mg daily
CoQ10	A nutrient most commonly in meat. Supports energy production, mitochondria and fertility.	100-200mg daily
B complex vitamin	A blend of B vitamins to support energy most commonly found in meat. Commonly depleted while taking metformin or birth control	One capsule daily

Root Gut Health Supplements:

The following are our most commonly used gut health supplements to support the gut health protocol steps: Remove, Replace, Repair, Reinocculate. We do not start a gut health supplement protocol if pregnant.

When starting the gut health protocol supplements, you can stagger start each new supplement by one week apart. This way you can make sure you are tolerating each supplement.

Remove:

Microbiome balance is a blend of herbs we use to rebalance the microbiome including gently removing overgrowth of bacteria in the small intestine. We find this a helpful first step for people experiencing bloating and/or constipation or loose stools. Our members typically only take this for 60 days.

Replace:

Digestive Enzymes can be helpful to support digestion and absorption of nutrients and healthy fats for hormone production and blood sugar balance. They are also helpful for those experiencing bloating after meals. When the gut is inflamed, our own digestive enzymes that are located in the inflamed lining of the gut, do not function optimally. We will typically support digestion with replacement for 3-6 months, depending on symptoms.

Repair:

Certain nutrients and herbs can help repair, soothe, and protect the single cell lining of the gut. We use a gut health powder called Gut Health Rebalance once a day, plus or minus Gut Health Protect, which is an immunoglobulin helpful especially in the presence of autoimmune disease like Hashimoto's. We use gut repair supplements for about 3 months, and then as needed if symptoms flare back up.

Reinoculate:

Reinoculate or repopulate good bacteria. Probiotics can certainly be tailored to the individual both with respect to strains and length of use. We typically use megaspore if bloating or acne are key issues. We then use a good well rounded probiotic with several strains in our Root probiotic, which is also shelf stable, but more cost effective for longer term use.

Microbiome Balance (Remove)	Blend of herbs to gently rebalance the microbiome if overgrowth is suspected	One capsule each morning before breakfast for one bottle.
Digestive Enzymes (Replace)	Supports the digestion of protein, fats, and carbs.	One capsule with a meal up to three times a day. For 3 months or as needed.
Gut Health Rebalance (Repair)	Nutrients and soothing herbs to support the gut lining. Helpful with heartburn as well.	One scoop dissolved in water daily. For 3 months or as desired.
Gut Health Protect (Repair)	Immunoglobulin. Helpful for binding toxins, protecting the lining of the gut. Also very helpful for diarrhea.	2-4 capsules daily for 3-6 months or as desired.
Megaspore (Reinoculate)	Probiotic	Follow directions on bottle. 3 months or as needed after this.
Root Probiotic (Reinoculate)	Probiotic	One daily. Maintenance probiotic

Symptom Survey

Instructions: Using the scale of symptom points listed below, fill in the appropriate score to the left of every symptom listed. Write the "Grand Total" at the top. If this is the initial symptom survey, Score every symptom based on your experience over the past month. If this is a follow up survey, score symptoms from the past week.

Scale of Symptom Points

If you did not suffer from the symptom ever or almost never, leave it blank.

1 = OCCASIONALLY (less than 2 times per week) and symptom was MILD
2 = FREQUENTLY (2 or more times per week) and symptom was MILD
3 = OCCASIONALLY (less than 2 times per week) and symptom was SEVERE
4 = FREQUENTLY (2 or more times per week) and symptom was SEVERE

```
┌─────────────────┐
│   Grand Total    │
│                  │
│                  │
└─────────────────┘
```

Constitutional		Nasal/Sinus		Musculoskeletal	
	Fatigue (sluggish, tired)		Post nasal drip		Join pain
	Restless (can't relax/sit still)		Sinus pain		Stiff joints
	Daytime sleepiness		Runny nose		Muscle aches/stiffness
	Insomnia at night		Stuffy nose		Muscle cramps
	Total		Sneezing		Total
Emotional/Mental			Total	**Cardiovascular**	
	Depression	**Mouth/Throat**			Racing or low heartbeat
	Anxiety (fears, uneasiness)		Sore or swollen throat		High blood pressure
	Mood swings (rapid changes)		Swelling/burning lips/tongue		Total
	Irritability		Throat clearing	**Digestive**	
	Forgetfulness		Canker sores		Heartburn/reflux
	Brain fog		Difficulty swallowing		Abdominal pain
	Low sex drive		Total		Constipation
	Total	**Lungs**			Diarrhea
Head/Ears			Wheezing		Painful bloating
	Headache (not migraine)		Cough		Gas
	Migraine		Shortness of breath		Nausea
	Earache		Total		Vomiting
	Jaw pain	**Eyes**			Total
	Ringing in ears		Red or swollen eyes	**Weight Management**	
	Discharge from ears/fluid in ears		Watery eyes		Fluctuating weight
	Itchy ears		Itchy eyes		Food cravings
	Sensitivity to sound		Sensitivity to light		Water retention
	Total		Total		Binge eating or drinking
Skin		**Genitourinary**			Total
	Blemishes, acne		Urinary frequency		
	Rashes or hives		Painful urination		
	Flushing of cheeks		Bladder pain		
	Itchy skin		Total		
	Total				

Chapter One

1. Epidemiology, diagnosis, and management of polycystic ovary syndrome (2014)
   1. https://www.ncbi.nlm.nih.gov/pmc/articles/PMC3872139/
2. Recent advances in the understanding and management of polycystic ovary syndrome (2019)
   1. https://www.ncbi.nlm.nih.gov/pmc/articles/PMC6489978/
3. Physiology, Thyroid Function (2021)
   1. https://www.ncbi.nlm.nih.gov/books/NBK537039/
4. Hashimoto Thyroiditis (2021)
   1. https://www.ncbi.nlm.nih.gov/books/NBK459262/
5. Mahan, L.K, Escott-Stump, S., Raymond, J.L. (2012). *Krause's Food and the Nutrition Care Process*. Elsevier Inc.
6. Autoimmune disease during pregnancy and the microchimerism legacy of pregnancy (2009)
   1. https://www.ncbi.nlm.nih.gov/pmc/articles/PMC2709983/
7. Thyroid disorders in polycystic ovarian syndrome subjects: a tertiary hospital based cross-sectional study from Eastern India (2013)
   1. https://pubmed.ncbi.nlm.nih.gov/23776908/
8. High prevalence of autoimmune thyroiditis in patients with polycystic ovary syndrome (2004)
   1. https://pubmed.ncbi.nlm.nih.gov/15012623/

9. Thyroid and fertility: recent advances (2020)

    1. https://pubmed.ncbi.nlm.nih.gov/31903865/

10. Pregnancy in polycystic ovary syndrome (2013)

    1. https://www.ncbi.nlm.nih.gov/pmc/articles/ PMC3659904/

Chapter Two

1. Epidemiology, diagnosis, and management of polycystic ovary syndrome (2014)

    1. https://www.ncbi.nlm.nih.gov/pmc/articles/ PMC3872139/

2. Oral contraceptives and changes in nutritional requirements (2013)

    1. https://pubmed.ncbi.nlm.nih.gov/23852908/

3. Hormonal contraception in women with polycystic ovary syndrome: choices, challenges, and noncontraceptive benefits (2017)

    1. https://www.ncbi.nlm.nih.gov/pmc/articles/ PMC5774551/

4. Treatment of infertility in women with polycystic ovary syndrome: approach to clinical practice (2015)

    1. https://www.ncbi.nlm.nih.gov/pmc/articles/ PMC4642490/

5. Long-term metformin use and vitamin B12 deficiency in the diabetes prevention program outcomes study (2016)

    1. https://www.ncbi.nlm.nih.gov/pmc/articles/ PMC4880159/

6. Multiple autoimmune syndrome (2010)

    1. https://www.ncbi.nlm.nih.gov/pmc/articles/ PMC3150011/

Chapter Three

1. Inflammatory markers in women with polycystic ovary syndrome (2020)

1. https://www.ncbi.nlm.nih.gov/pmc/articles/
   PMC7079227/
2. Debates regarding lean patients with polycystic ovary syndrome: a narrative review (2017)
   1. https://www.ncbi.nlm.nih.gov/pmc/articles/
      PMC5672719/
3. Epidemiology, diagnosis, and management of polycystic ovary syndrome (2014)
   1. https://www.ncbi.nlm.nih.gov/pmc/articles/
      PMC3872139/
4. Studies of insulin resistance in patients with clinical and sub-clinical hypothyroidism (2009)
   1. https://pubmed.ncbi.nlm.nih.gov/19141606/
5. A comparative study on insulin secretion, insulin resistance and thyroid function in patients with polycystic ovary syndrome with and without Hashimoto's thyroiditis (2021)
   1. https://pubmed.ncbi.nlm.nih.gov/33953581/
6. Thyroid-stimulating hormone is associated with insulin resistance independently of body mass index and age in women with polycystic ovary syndrome (2009)
   1. https://pubmed.ncbi.nlm.nih.gov/19654109/
7. Role of gut microbiota in the development of insulin resistance and the mechanism underlying polycystic ovary syndrome: a review (2020)
   1. https://www.ncbi.nlm.nih.gov/pmc/articles/
      PMC7301991/
8. Thyroid-gut-axis: how does the microbiota influence thyroid function? (2020)
   1. https://www.ncbi.nlm.nih.gov/pmc/articles/
      PMC7353203/

Chapter Four

1. The pathogenesis of polycystic ovary syndrome (PCOS): the hypothesis of PCOS as functional ovarian hyperandrogenism revisited (2016)
   1. https://www.ncbi.nlm.nih.gov/pmc/articles/PMC5045492/
2. Hyperandrogenism in polycystic ovarian syndrome and role of CYP gene variants: a review (2019)
   1. https://jmhg.springeropen.com/articles/10.1186/s43042-019-0031-4
3. The polycystic ovary syndrome: an update on metabolic and hormonal mechanisms (2015)
   1. https://www.ncbi.nlm.nih.gov/pmc/articles/PMC4392092/
4. High prevalence of Hashimoto's thyroiditis in patients with polycystic ovary syndrome: does the imbalance between estradiol and progesterone play a role? (2015)
   1. https://pubmed.ncbi.nlm.nih.gov/25822940/

Chapter Five

1. The adrenal and polycystic ovary syndrome (2007)
   1. https://pubmed.ncbi.nlm.nih.gov/17932770/
2. Stress-related development of obesity and cortisol in women (2009)
   1. https://www.ncbi.nlm.nih.gov/pubmed/19300426
3. Serum cortisol level variations in thyroid diseases (2000)
   1. https://pubmed.ncbi.nlm.nih.gov/14666786/
4. Elevated thyroid stimulating hormone is associated with elevated cortisol in healthy young men and women (2012)
   1. https://www.ncbi.nlm.nih.gov/pmc/articles/PMC3520819/
5. Stress and thyroid autoimmunity (2004)
   1. https://pubmed.ncbi.nlm.nih.gov/15650357/

6. Dried urine and salivary profiling for complete assessment of cortisol and cortisol metabolites (2020)
   1. https://www.sciencedirect.com/science/article/pii/S221462372030096X
7. Stress management in women with Hashimoto's thyroiditis: a randomized controlled trial (2019)
   1. https://www.ncbi.nlm.nih.gov/pmc/articles/PMC6688766/

Chapter Six
1. Polycystic ovary syndrome and mitochondrial dysfunction (2019)
   1. https://www.ncbi.nlm.nih.gov/pmc/articles/PMC6698037/
2. The relationship between oxidative stress and autoimmunity in Hashimoto's thyroiditis (2015)
   1. https://pubmed.ncbi.nlm.nih.gov/26340971/
3. Pregnancy in polycystic ovary syndrome (2013)
   1. https://www.ncbi.nlm.nih.gov/pmc/articles/PMC3659904/
4. Oxidative stress as a key feature of autoimmune thyroiditis: an update (2020)
   1. https://pubmed.ncbi.nlm.nih.gov/32969631/
5. Influence of dietary habits on oxidative stress markers in Hashimoto's thyroiditis (2021)
   1. https://pubmed.ncbi.nlm.nih.gov/32729374/
6. Oxidative stress and BPA toxicity: an antioxidant approach for male and female reproductive dysfunction (2020)
   1. https://pubmed.ncbi.nlm.nih.gov/32397641/
7. Meta-analysis of association between between vitamin D and autoimmune thyroid disease (2015)
   1. https://pubmed.ncbi.nlm.nih.gov/25854833/
8. The effects of vitamin D supplementation on biomarkers of inflammation and oxidative stress among women with polycystic

ovary syndrome: a systematic review and meta-analysis of randomized controlled trials (2018)

    1. https://pubmed.ncbi.nlm.nih.gov/29475212/

9. Mitochondrial (dys)function and insulin resistance: from pathophysiological molecular mechanisms to the impact of diet (2019)

    1. https://www.ncbi.nlm.nih.gov/pmc/articles/
       PMC6510277/

Chapter Seven

1. Role of gut microbiota in the development of insulin resistance and the mechanism underlying polycystic ovary syndrome: a review (2020)

    1. https://www.ncbi.nlm.nih.gov/pmc/articles/
       PMC7301991/

2. Thyroid-Gut-Axis: How does the microbiota influence thyroid function? (2020)

    1. https://www.ncbi.nlm.nih.gov/pmc/articles/
       PMC7353203/

3. Serum zonulin is elevated in women with PCOS and correlates with insulin resistance and severity of anovulation (2015)

    1. https://pubmed.ncbi.nlm.nih.gov/25336505/

4. Is eating behavior manipulated by the gastrointestinal microbiota? Evolutionary pressures and potential mechanisms (2014)

    1. https://pubmed.ncbi.nlm.nih.gov/25103109/

5. Exploration of the relationship between gut microbiota and polycystic ovary syndrome (PCOS): a review (2020)

    1. https://www.ncbi.nlm.nih.gov/pmc/articles/
       PMC7035130/

6. Estrogen-gut microbiome axis: physiological and clinical implications (2017)

    1. https://pubmed.ncbi.nlm.nih.gov/28778332/

7. Thyroid-Gut-Axis: How does the microbiota influence thyroid function? (2020)

1. https://www.ncbi.nlm.nih.gov/pmc/articles/
   PMC7353203/

8. Link between hypothyroidism and small intestinal bacterial over-growth (2014)
   1. https://www.ncbi.nlm.nih.gov/pmc/articles/
      PMC4056127/

Chapter Eight

1. The effectiveness of intermittent fasting to reduce body mass index and glucose metabolism: a systematic review and meta-analysis (2019)
   1. https://www.ncbi.nlm.nih.gov/pubmed/31601019
2. Fasting as possible complementary approach for polycystic ovary syndrome: hope or hype? (2017)
   1. https://pubmed.ncbi.nlm.nih.gov/28735644/
3. Eight-hour time-restricted feeding improves endocrine and metabolic profiles in women with anovulatory polycystic ovary syndrome (2021)
   1. https://pubmed.ncbi.nlm.nih.gov/17374948/
4. Effectiveness of myoinositol for polycystic ovary syndrome: a systematic review and meta-analysis (2017)
   1. https://pubmed.ncbi.nlm.nih.gov/29052180/
5. Treatment with myo-inositol and selenium ensures euthyroidism in patients with autoimmune thyroiditis (2017)
   1. https://www.ncbi.nlm.nih.gov/pmc/articles/
      PMC5331475/
6. Myo-inositol plus selenium supplementation restores euthyroid state in Hashimoto's patients with subclinical hypothyroidism (2017)
   1. https://pubmed.ncbi.nlm.nih.gov/28724185/
7. Insulin sensitiser agents alone and in co-treatment with r-FSH for ovulation induction in PCOS women (2010)
   1. https://pubmed.ncbi.nlm.nih.gov/20222840/

8. Clinical, endocrine and metabolic effects of metformin vs N-acetyl-cysteine in women with polycystic ovary syndrome (2011)
    1. https://pubmed.ncbi.nlm.nih.gov/21831508/
9. A comparison between the effects of metformin and N-acetyl cysteine (NAC) on some metabolic and endocrine characteristics of women with polycystic ovary syndrome (2016)
    1. https://pubmed.ncbi.nlm.nih.gov/26654154/
10. A review on various uses of N-acetyl cysteine (2017)
    1. https://www.ncbi.nlm.nih.gov/pmc/articles/PMC5241507/
11. Mitochondrial (dys)function and insulin resistance: from patho-physiological molecular mechanisms to the impact of diet (2019)
    1. https://www.ncbi.nlm.nih.gov/pmc/articles/PMC6510277/
12. Effectiveness of omega-3 fatty acid for polycystic ovary syndrome: a systematic review and meta-analysis (2018)
    1. https://www.ncbi.nlm.nih.gov/pmc/articles/PMC5870911/
13. The effects of vitamin D supplementation on biomarkers of inflammation and oxidative stress among women with polycystic ovary syndrome: a systematic review and meta-analysis of randomized controlled trials (2018)
    1. https://pubmed.ncbi.nlm.nih.gov/29475212/
14. Effects of zinc supplementation on markers of insulin resistance and lipid profiles in women with polycystic ovary syndrome: a randomized, double-blind, placebo-controlled trial (2015)
    1. https://pubmed.ncbi.nlm.nih.gov/25868059/
15. Effects of zinc supplementation on endocrine outcomes in women with polycystic ovary syndrome: a randomized, double-blind, placebo-controlled trial (2016)
    1. https://pubmed.ncbi.nlm.nih.gov/26315303/
16. Prevalence of celiac disease in patients with autoimmune thyroid disease: a meta-analysis (2016)

   1. https://pubmed.ncbi.nlm.nih.gov/27256300/

17. Celiac disease and autoimmune thyroid disease (2007)
   1. https://www.ncbi.nlm.nih.gov/pmc/articles/ PMC2111403/

18. The effect of gluten-free diet on thyroid autoimmunity in drug-naive women with Hashimoto's thyroiditis: a pilot study (2019)
   1. https://pubmed.ncbi.nlm.nih.gov/30060266/

19. The importance of nutritional factors and dietary management of Hashimoto's thyroiditis (2020)
   1. https://pubmed.ncbi.nlm.nih.gov/32588591/

20. A prospective study of dairy foods intake and anovulatory infertility (2007)
   1. https://pubmed.ncbi.nlm.nih.gov/17329264/

21. Decrease in TSH levels after lactose restriction in Hashimoto's thyroiditis patients with lactose intolerance (2014)
   1. https://pubmed.ncbi.nlm.nih.gov/24078411/

22. Effect of soy phytoestrogen on metabolic and hormonal disturbance of women with polycystic ovary syndrome (2011)
   1. https://www.ncbi.nlm.nih.gov/pmc/articles/ PMC3214337/

23. The effects of soy isoflavones on metabolic status of patients with polycystic ovary syndrome (2016)
   1. https://pubmed.ncbi.nlm.nih.gov/27490918/

24. Impact of short-term isoflavone intervention in polycystic ovary syndrome (PCOS) patients on microbiota composition and metagenomics (2020)
   1. https://pubmed.ncbi.nlm.nih.gov/32492805/

25. The effect of soy phytoestrogen supplementation on thyroid status and cardiovascular risk markers in patients with subclinical hypothyroidism: a randomized, double-blind, crossover study (2011)
   1. https://pubmed.ncbi.nlm.nih.gov/21325465/

26. Effects of dietary phytoestrogens on hormones throughout the human lifespan: a review (2020)
   1. https://pubmed.ncbi.nlm.nih.gov/32824177/
27. Time- and dose-dependent effects of roundup on human embryonic and placental cells (2007)
   1. https://pubmed.ncbi.nlm.nih.gov/17486286/
28. Assessment of glyphosate induced epigenetic transgenerational inheritance of pathologies and sperm epimutations: generational toxicology (2019)
   1. https://pubmed.ncbi.nlm.nih.gov/31011160/
29. The Ramazzini Institute 13-week pilot study on glyphosate and Roundup administered at human-equivalent dose to Sprague Dawley rats: effects on the microbiome (2018)
   1. https://pubmed.ncbi.nlm.nih.gov/29843725/

Chapter Nine
   1. A review of zinc-l-carnosine and its positive effects on oral mucositis, taste disorders, and gastrointestinal disorders (2020)
      1. https://www.ncbi.nlm.nih.gov/pmc/articles/PMC7146259/
   2. The roles of glutamine in the intestine and its implication in intestinal diseases (2017)
      1. https://www.ncbi.nlm.nih.gov/pmc/articles/PMC5454963/
   3. *Bacillus* supp. Spores—a promising treatment option for patients with irritable bowel syndrome (2019)
      1. https://www.ncbi.nlm.nih.gov/pmc/articles/PMC6770835/
   4. Oral spore-based probiotic supplementation was associated with reduced incidence of post-prandial dietary endotoxin, triglycerides, and disease risk biomarkers (2017)
      1. https://pubmed.ncbi.nlm.nih.gov/28868181/

5. The effect of probiotic *Bacillus subtilis* HU58 on immune function in healthy human (2017)

    1. https://journals.indexcopernicus.com/api/file/viewByFileId/602370.pdf

6. Investigating the role of perceived stress on bacterial flora activity and salivary cortisol secretion: a possible mechanism underlying susceptibility to illness (2008).

    1. https://pubmed.ncbi.nlm.nih.gov/18023961/

Chapter Ten

1. Depression, anxiety and perceived stress in women with and without PCOS: a community-based study (2019)

    1. https://pubmed.ncbi.nlm.nih.gov/30131078/

2. Psychological distress in women with polycystic ovary syndrome from Imam Khomeini Hospital, Tehran (2012)

    1. https://www.ncbi.nlm.nih.gov/pmc/articles/PMC3719335/

3. High prevalence of moderate and severe depressive and anxiety symptoms in polycystic ovary syndrome: a systematic review and meta-analysis (2017)

    1. https://pubmed.ncbi.nlm.nih.gov/28333286/

4. Hyperandrogenism in polycystic ovarian syndrome and role of CYP gene variants: a review (2019)

    1. https://jmhg.springeropen.com/articles/10.1186/s43042-019-0031-4

5. Mindfulness-based stress reduction for healthy individuals : a meta-analysis (2015)

    1. https://pubmed.ncbi.nlm.nih.gov/25818837/

6. Impact of a mindfulness stress management program on stress, anxiety, depression and quality of life in women with polycystic ovary syndrome: a randomized controlled trial (2015)

    1. https://pubmed.ncbi.nlm.nih.gov/25287137/

7. Cognitive-behavioral therapy improves weight loss and quality of life in women with polycystic ovary syndrome: a pilot randomized clinical trial (2018)
   1. https://pubmed.ncbi.nlm.nih.gov/29908771/
8. Sleep disturbances in women with polycystic ovary syndrome: prevalence, pathophysiology, impact, and management strategies (2018)
   1. https://www.ncbi.nlm.nih.gov/pmc/articles/ PMC5799701/
9. An alternative treatment for anxiety: a systematic review of human trial results reported for the Ayurvedic herb ashwagandha (*Withania somnifera*) (2014)
   1. https://www.ncbi.nlm.nih.gov/pmc/articles/ PMC4270108/
10. An investigation into the stress-relieving and pharmacological actions of an ashwagandha (*Withania somnifera*) extract (2019)
    1. https://www.ncbi.nlm.nih.gov/pmc/articles/ PMC6750292/
11. Efficacy and safety of ashwagandha root extract in subclinical hypothyroid patients: a double-blind, randomized placebo-controlled trial (2018)
    1. https://pubmed.ncbi.nlm.nih.gov/28829155/
12. Ethnobiology and ethnopharmacology of *Lepidium meyenii* (maca), a plant from the Peruvian highlands (2012)
    1. https://www.ncbi.nlm.nih.gov/pmc/articles/ PMC3184420/
13. GABA and L-theanine mixture decreases sleep latency and improves NREM sleep (2019)
    1. https://www.ncbi.nlm.nih.gov/pmc/articles/ PMC6366437/
14. The effects of magnesium supplementation on subjective anxiety and stress—a systematic review (2017)

1. https://www.ncbi.nlm.nih.gov/pmc/articles/
   PMC5452159/

www.ingramcontent.com/pod-product-compliance
Lightning Source LLC
Chambersburg PA
CBHW050238270326
41914CB00034BA/1965/J